CARING IN AN AGE OF REFORM

A HISTORY OF GUY'S AND ST THOMAS' 1948 TO 2010

STEPHANIE J SNOW

Editing, design, typesetting and publishing by UK Book Publishing.

www.ukbookpublishing.com

ISBN: 978-1-917329-08-8

In recognition of all Guy's and St Thomas' patients, staff and alumni – past, present and future

Contents

e

Acknowledgements

T his book has been a long time in the making, and I am hugely grateful for the patience and understanding of the many people who contributed to the work, and to the Guy's and St Thomas' Charity who funded the research. From the outset, Guy's and St Thomas' communities of patients, staff, and alumni have been tremendously supportive and encouraging, giving time and energy in so many different ways. Most striking has been the strong, collective desire and willingness to reflect on and learn from the past. Without the generosity of people sharing their memories, reflections, and insights, alongside personal papers and photographs, it simply would not have been possible to create a history that bears witness to the vitality, strength, and compassion of these communities.

The idea for a Guy's and St Thomas' History Project originated from Bryan McSwiney who served as the 23rd and final Clerk of the Governors at St Thomas' between 1962 and 1974. Bryan continued his association with St Thomas', becoming Administrator of the Special Trustees for St Thomas' Hospital and Chair of the Veterans' Association. Bryan's enthusiasm led to the setting up of a Steering Group of alumni across Guy's and St Thomas' including Cyril Chantler, Bob Nicholls, Mike O'Brien, John Wyn Owen and Richard Sawyer, who were joined by Patricia Moberly, then Chairman of Guy's and St Thomas' Foundation Trust. The Group secured initial support from the Guy's and St Thomas' Charity to hold a Witness Seminar in 2011 and I was appointed to lead the work. Following the Witness Seminar we were awarded a further grant which sustained the interviews and archival work between 2012 and 2015. During the research period, the work benefited enormously from the advice and support of an Advisory Group including Ron Kerr, then Chief

Executive, Patricia Moberly, then Chairman, Cyril Chantler, Anne-Marie Rafferty, Stephen Jenkins, Geoffrey Rivett and Rick Trainor.

Many historians shy away from commissioned histories because of the difficulties in reconciling the institution's desire and expectation that the historical output will amplify the positive at the expense of the historian's task of giving equal account to difficult aspects and events. I was extremely grateful that because of the exemplary leadership of Patricia Moberly, these dilemmas were avoided. During the initial Witness Seminar, Patricia set out the boundaries: 'Once we've secured more funding, the Steering Group will have no further remit and no editorial control and the project will be totally in the hands of the professional team.' She remained true to her word and although the Advisory Group was extremely supportive whilst the research was being conducted, Patricia decided that it would not be appropriate for the Group to comment on or see drafts of the book in advance of the final publication. Patricia died in 2016 and there have also been other sad losses of interviewees including Peter Lumsden, Brian Marchant and John Wyn Owen. This is not unexpected given the age range of contributors, but it emphasises the value of a project of this sort which captures people's reflections and experiences and with interviewees' permission, preserves them as a legacy for the benefit of future research.

I am very grateful for the assistance of archivists at the London Metropolitan Archives, the National Archives, King's College London Archives and the Wellcome Collection. Many interviewees shared their personal papers and photographs, which was tremendously helpful for developing the most rounded view of events, and these individuals are listed in the Sources section. For their help in sourcing images and securing permissions I thank Bill Edwards, Curator at the Gordon Museum, and Penelope Hines at Guy's and St Thomas' Charity. I would particularly like to thank the late Brian Marchant's family who gave me permission to use one of the photographs that

Brian shared at the time of his interview as the cover illustration. During the research period I was fortunate to have the assistance of Julian Simpson who undertook much of the archive work and interviews. Special thanks go to Erin Beeston who provided superb support and skills through drafting chapters; and Michael Lambert who undertook a rigorous review of a full draft of the book that saved me from blunders and helped strengthen it further. I am also very grateful to the interviewees who have responded to my follow-up queries and checked drafts for accuracy. Any remaining errors of fact or misunderstandings remain mine alone.

Throughout the research and the long period of writing I have benefited from discussions with colleagues, and feedback on seminar and conference papers. This has added richness and depth to the work and I thank you all, especially Kath Checkland, Anna Coleman, Martin Gorsky, Jennifer Gunn, Peter Kernahan, Imelda McDermott, Graham Moody, Sally Sheard, Elizabeth Toon and Jo Van Every. On many occasions the creation of this book has become a family activity, so finally but most importantly, I thank David, Evie, Verity and Gwyn for their enduring love and support.

List of figures and illustrations

Figures

Illustrations

8. Renal nursing education session underway at the Renal Unit, Lambeth Hospital c.1970s © Marianne Vennegoor.

9. Jack Tulley, Professor of Orthodontics and Dean 1980-1985, teaching dental students at Guy's c. late 1970s/early 1980s © Gordon Museum, King's College London.

10. Brian Marchant, dialysis patient at St Thomas', c.1970 © Brian Marchant. (also used on front book cover)

11. Medicine across the generations: Richard Hughes, Emeritus Professor of Neurology, Guy's, holding a portrait of Robert Hughes his great grandfather who was also a Guy's alumnus © Julian Simpson.

12. Natalie Tiddy, Nightingale Nurse c.1960s © Natalie Tiddy.

13. Celebrations in Guy's courtyard c.1980s © Gordon Museum, King's College London.

14. 30 years of service: Mike Messer (right) and colleagues at the St Thomas' Medical School, Annual Sports Day c.1970s © Mike Messer

15. Mike Messer (right) and colleagues at a dinner to mark the end of teaching in Block Nine, St Thomas' c.2000s © Mike Messer.

16. Spoof site plan created during the merger of Guy's and St Thomas' NHS Trusts, c.1990s.

17. Campaign poster for Save Guy's and St Thomas' Hospitals c.1990s © Marianne Vennegoor.

18. Christopher Bramaje and Cecilia Saquing at work, Guy's and St Thomas' NHS Foundation Trust, 2014 © Julian Simpson.

19. Abdul Chowdhury, chaplain, Guy's and St Thomas' NHS Foundation Trust, 2013 © Julian Simpson.

20. South Wing Corridor, St Thomas' Hospital c.1900 and 2007 © Mike Messer

21. Commissioned for the millennium this piece symbolises the relationships of trust and help that exist between patient and healer, and the joining together of Guy's and St Thomas' hospitals. Cross the Divide, 2000 © Rick Kirby. (also used on back book cover)

22. Guy's Campus, King's College London, 2013 © Julian Simpson.

23. Rainbow badge initiated by Dr Michael Farquhar, consultant, Evelina London, 2019 © Michael Farquhar.

Sources and abbreviations

Sources

KCL	King's College London Archives
LMA	London Metropolitan Archives, London
TNA	The National Archives, Kew, London
WT	Wellcome Collection, London

Private sources

KC	Karen Caines
SCF	Sandra Carnall Ferrelly
SC	Stephen Challacombe
CC	Cyril Chantler
WLD	Wyndham Lloyd-Davies
MG	Mike Gleeson
TH	Tania Herniman
RH	Richard Hughes
JJ	Joachim Jose
JL	John Lister
KL	Kay Lucey
BM	Brian Marchant
MM	Mike Messer
PMob	Patricia Moberly
BM	Betsy Morley
PM	Patricia Mowbray
BN	Bob Nicholls
JWO	John Wyn Owen
CR	Carol Rowe
RS	Richard Sawyer

LS   Lee Soden
BS   Barbara Stevens
NT   Natalie Tiddy
MV   Marianne Vennegoor
TY   Tony Young

Interviews

Group interviews focused on four specific areas of interest were undertaken: budgets; catering; faith; and training. These involved 17 interviewees. Individual interviews were conducted with 80 interviewees. The name of the interviewee and the date of the interview are given in the notes. Several interviewees requested to remain anonymous and they have been allocated a unique identifying number.

CHAPTER ONE

Introduction

From their beginnings, Guy's and St Thomas' hospitals and associated institutions have been principal players in the local, national, and international landscape of medicine and healthcare. The discoveries and innovations made by alumni include blood transfusions using human blood; intraocular lens surgery for cataracts; tissue typing; and kidney transplants to name just a few. The figurehead of modern nursing, Florence Nightingale, set up her nursing school at St Thomas' in 1860, and in 2016, a statue of Mary Seacole, described as a pathfinder for the generations of National Health Service (NHS) staff from ethnically diverse backgrounds was installed in the garden at St Thomas'.[1] Innovation has stretched beyond medicine and nursing. A bleep system invented by Peter Styles in 1953 at St Thomas' revolutionised hospital working practices worldwide. Guy's successfully pioneered the introduction of clinical directorates to the UK in 1985. Guy's and St Thomas' was the first Trust to introduce the wearing of Rainbow Badges in the 2010s which were initiated by Dr Michael Farquhar, consultant at Evelina Children's Hospital, to raise awareness of LGBTQ+ issues and challenge negative attitudes towards LGBTQ+ people. Most recently, Guy's and St Thomas' are working with other hospital trusts and charities on a programme for patient, carer, and public involvement in Covid-19 recovery. Funded by Guy's and St Thomas' Charity and King's College Hospital Charity, the work involves co-designing with patients, a holistic, evidence-based treatment pathway to ensure that people living with long Covid-19 get the very best of care.[2]

Since becoming part of the NHS in 1948, the size and the complexity of Guy's and St Thomas' – hospitals, medical, nursing, dental schools, academic health sciences centre – and their integrated functions of care, research, and teaching has led them to play a central role in the evolution of the NHS and healthcare more broadly. The first reorganisation of the NHS in 1974 accorded them new responsibilities for services for local populations; Guy's and Lewisham NHS Trust was the flagship trust for the introduction of the quasi-market to the NHS in 1991; and opposition to the merger of Guy's and St Thomas' hospitals provoked public campaigns and petitions with more than 1,000 signatories. Guy's and St Thomas' have also shaped the reconfiguration of medical education and the rationalisation of hospital care in London which were driven by wider influences such as the shift to integrate medicine within the broader academic context of a university and the move towards supra-specialist services.

Operating across the southeast London boroughs of Lambeth, Southwark, and Lewisham, Guy's and St Thomas' patient populations are drawn from some of the most deprived areas of the UK with significant inequalities in health. London has long been recognised as an area which presents major challenges for healthcare provision on account of the volume and density of its population, the range and diversity of individuals, and the extremes of wealth and poverty within one geographical area. The broad features of London are heightened in the southeast London boroughs under Guy's and St Thomas' care which have patient populations with higher-than-average needs and, since the 1960s, growing multi-ethnic communities. St Thomas' introduced new initiatives such as shared care in obstetrics and diabetes, and developed Lambeth Community Care Centre as a community hospital in the 1970s. Services have also been created to meet the health needs of specific ethnic groups such as the African Well Women's Clinic, set up by Guy's midwife Comfort Momoh in 1997 to care for women affected by female genital mutilation (FGM).

Alongside providing care for local patients, Guy's and St Thomas' have also stood as international centres, taking patients from all parts of the world for rare and specialist treatments.

London's skylines and panoramas are defined by the institutions' buildings. Guy's Tower, opened in 1974 as the tallest hospital building in the world, now blending with the seventeenth century dome of St Paul's cathedral and newer icons of the Shard and the Gherkin. Refurbished in the late 2000s, it has now reclaimed its world status for height thanks to the installation of a sculpture by German artist, Carsten Nicolai, which at night casts moving beams of light across the capital.[3] Looking across the river Thames to the Houses of Parliament and Big Ben, St Thomas' hospital site, now housing the A&E department of Guy's and St Thomas', is the strongest material evidence of the institutions' long and tight connections to the centres of political, medical, and institutional power. It is frequently described in the media as 'the politicians' hospital' and indeed, cared for the former Prime Minister, Boris Johnson, when he was acutely ill with Covid-19 in spring 2020. Close links to the seats of power have often resulted in the institutions being at the vanguard of change and early adopters of new policies. The Chief Executive and the General Manager of Guy's and Lewisham NHS Trust had been civil servants who had played central roles in the development of policies around Trusts.[4] Appointments of medical staff to the Royal Medical Household and presidencies of the Royal Colleges have ensured that the institutions have enjoyed influence and agency. In 2019, Amanda Pritchard, Chief Executive of Guy's and St Thomas' since 2016, was appointed Chief Operating Officer for NHS England and in 2021 became NHS England's first female chief executive.

Since the 1970s Guy's and St Thomas' have become one institution through a succession of mergers of teaching institutions and hospitals, and the story of how and why this happened is the focus for this book. From the outside in Guy's and St Thomas' have more similarities than differences: elite transnational institutions, eminent past and present staff, generous endowment funds, and similar scopes of services and work. But for patients, staff, and local communities, the culture of each institution created a sharply differentiated identity which has been understood as central to the very way in which doctors practised medicine, nurses cared for patients, porters met ambulances, and food was prepared for patients. The chapters that follow explore this natural history, beginning with the creation of the NHS in 1948 and establishing the individual institutional histories before the definitive merger of the hospitals in 1993. The processes through which the institutions developed a new shared culture are evaluated, concluding with the creation of the Academic Health Sciences Centre in 2009.

Sources and methods

The main sources for the book are a Witness Seminar held in 2011, and oral history interviews carried out between 2011 and 2015 with 97 patients, staff, and other informants who have been associated with Guy's and St Thomas'. Oral evidence has been supported by archival material, interviewees' personal papers, and written contributions from other informants.[5] This has created a diverse range of perspectives which cut across the strata of the institutions and the different aspects of care, research, and teaching, reflecting variation and uniformity in experiences. Contributions include those from individuals who worked only briefly at Guy's and St Thomas' alongside those who stayed for decades. This approach has deepened the complexity of the analysis but importantly has captured something of the multifaceted and contingent nature of changes and continuities in healthcare over the period. Most interviewees have had experiences of work or care beyond Guy's and St Thomas', and this has enabled them to produce insights and comparisons that both sharpen the distinctiveness of Guy's and St Thomas', and help contextualise its history within the wider context of British healthcare.

Oral history is the most sensitive methodology for exploring experiences of life and work.[6] It has particular potency in an institutional setting as it captures not just the personal accounts of interviewees but illuminates the narratives embedded in the collective memory of the institutions.[7] The common feature that brings together generations and groupings of interviewees who have worked at Guy's and St Thomas' is the deep engagement with its core functions: the care of patients, the pursuit of scientific and medical knowledge, and the teaching of students. What good care, good research, and good teaching looked like varies across the period, taking different forms at different times. Nevertheless, the sense of striving towards a common purpose has held fast across time in Guy's and St Thomas', despite being severely weakened by mergers, and manifests itself most vibrantly in the metaphor of a family. The idea of a family – a close unit bound by common ties and emotional bonds – is often used by staff to describe their association with an organisation.[8] There have been multiple significant shifts across the period in Guy's and St Thomas', in working relationships and practices, ethnicity and gender of staff and patients, and many instances where individual experiences have been traumatic and uncomfortable. Yet the conviction that these interactions have taken place within a family has held fast across the generations and are expressed as strongly by current working staff as by earlier generations who are now retired. The consistency in the use of family as a metaphor for working life means that it cannot be dismissed as a nostalgia for a past, golden age. As in our wider society, the definition of a family in 2024 is very different to what it was in the 1970s. But it does suggest how common values and norms of behaviour that constitute local cultures have been transmitted through the generations of patients, staff, and publics and, over time, been renegotiated and reinterpreted to reflect wider social changes.

Indeed, the strong attachment of alumni, staff, and patients to Guy's and St Thomas' may be one of the reasons for the overwhelming support this study has received from potential participants. One caveat is that staff or patients who have had difficult or unpleasant experiences through their associations with the institutions would be unlikely to volunteer their contribution to this study. Some reassurance can be derived from the fact that interviewees have expressed strong criticisms at many levels from the broad political philosophies to the day-to-day running of the institutions. The use of interviews and documentary sources has been complementary. Interviews have sometimes undone narratives in official discourse and archival evidence has brought to the fore issues that are marginalised in interviews. The study has also been strengthened by access to interviewees' personal papers and written contributions from other informants whom we did not have the time or resources to interview.

Outline

The chapters are loosely divided into decades to give a chronological structure to the history. Chapter 2 begins with the creation of the NHS in 1948 and the move of Guy's and St Thomas' hospitals into a nationalised hospital system. Becoming part of the NHS gave the hospitals significant financial security and at the same time, the retention of the endowment funds and direct lines of communication to the Ministry of Health enabled them to maintain autonomy over developments. The period saw an important shift towards the hospitals taking on more responsibility for meeting the health needs of their local population alongside caring for patients, teaching medical students, and conducting clinical research. From the 1970s there were intensive political, scientific, and social changes that reshaped the NHS and had significant impact on Guy's and St Thomas', and these are explored in Chapter 3. The first reorganisation of NHS structures in 1974 was a watermark in the governance of all

UK teaching hospitals through the loss of the boards of governors and new accountability to the local health authority. For Guy's and St Thomas', it brought new responsibilities for service provision to local communities. More broadly, the growing costs of the NHS in the context of an ageing population and terrific expansion in medical technologies were producing 'dilemmas of choice' that forced the institutions to engage with the application of economic principles to health service management.[9] The new focus on funding and resource management led to the formation of a Resource Allocation Working Party in 1976 which produced a new formula for distributing funding across the NHS according to need rather than historical patterns, and this led to budget cuts for Guy's and St Thomas'. Chapter 4 recounts how Guy's and St Thomas' responded to the increasing financial pressures of the 1980s through the introduction of business models for the management and delivery of health services. It was a time of radical change across Guy's and St Thomas', and in 1983, Guy's and St Thomas' medical and dental schools merged to create the United Medical and Dental School (UMDS) followed by the merging of the nursing schools in the context of *Project 2000* which established an academic basis for nurse training in 1991. The chapter concludes with the hospitals becoming self-governing NHS trusts through the reforms introduced in the 1989 White Paper, *Working for Patients*. The 1990s stands as the most tumultuous decade in the longer history of Guy's and St Thomas'. As part of the wider reconfiguration of London health services, Guy's and St Thomas' newly-formed NHS Trusts were merged. Chapter 5 explores the merger process in detail and the slow and painful journey through which the institutions brought services together and began building a new culture of care. During the same period, UMDS and King's College merged medical and dental schools so that for the first time, medical and dental education was carried out within a multi-faculty institution. This is the subject of Chapter 6, alongside an account of the creation of Guy's and St Thomas' Charity through the merger of the Special Trustees of each institution. Chapter 7 describes how the 2000s saw Guy's and St Thomas' become one of the first NHS foundation trusts with a new leadership team focused on creating a more open and diverse institution that better reflected the local patient population and addressed longstanding tensions around hierarchies and closed cultures. The decade ended with the award of an Academic Health Sciences Centre to King's Health Partners, an achievement that could not have happened without the earlier, painful mergers of hospitals and teaching schools. The final chapter concludes by discussing the changes and continuities in the everyday experiences of students, patients, and staff since the 1970s. It reviews how Guy's and St Thomas' has maintained strong connections with the past despite the profound transformations across many aspects of institutional life and healthcare, and thus counters traditional narratives of radical linear change across the NHS. Institutional history is shown to be a vibrant and embedded influence across Guy's and St Thomas' which has the capacity to promote resilience and constancy to core values in the face of external flux and change.

CHAPTER TWO

Guy's, St Thomas', and the Early Years of the National Health Service, 1948–1970

Overview

The creation of the National Health Service (NHS) in 1948 marked a significant turning point in Guy's and St Thomas' longer institutional histories as their hospitals became part of a nationalised hospital system. Government funding provided welcome relief from the challenges of self-financing the hospitals. The institutions continued to be overseen by reconfigured Boards of Governors and had direct lines of communication to the Ministry of Health. These arrangements, alongside the retention of control over the endowment funds, allowed Guy's and St Thomas' to maintain autonomy over institutional developments through to the 1970s. The importance of the 1948 to 1974 period in the history of the NHS has been generally underplayed by historians due to the heavy focus placed on NHS reform through structural and functional reorganisations which began in 1974. In fact, this was a key period of innovation across all aspects of healthcare. Hospital sites were rebuilt and upgraded to support the development of new services and treatments. The increasing complexity of healthcare organisation required more sophisticated management arrangements. Less visible but equally significant change was taking place in redirecting the focus of these historic teaching hospitals on to the health needs of local populations across Southwark, Lambeth, and Lewisham.

Origins

The history of Guy's and St Thomas' hospitals and associated institutions is long and deeply intertwined; St Thomas' has its origins in the twelfth century and Guy's was created in the 1700s specifically to care for patients not eligible to be treated at St Thomas'. As Guy's was viewed 'as a kind of annexe or extension to St Thomas', with common rather than rival interests', there was no initial rivalry between the hospitals.[1] Students could avail themselves of teaching and learning opportunities at both medical schools and hospitals. In 1769, surgical and medical teaching were split between the hospitals, the former at St Thomas', the latter at Guy's, and the schools became known as the United Hospitals of the Borough. This partnership continued until 1825, when a dispute over the appointment of a successor to Guy's surgeon, Sir Astley Cooper, led to the creation of an independent medical school under the direction of Guy's Hospital.[2] The United Friends Hospitals Dining Club was established in 1828 to preserve friendly relations and students continued to attend surgical operations at both institutions. In 1836, however, a student riot in St Thomas' operating theatre led to a complete separation, despite the institutions remaining in physical proximity to each other for another 30 or so years. Both operated as voluntary hospitals relying on philanthropic contributions and were managed by lay Boards of Governors, with physicians and surgeons holding honorary posts. From this point onwards, the differences between Guy's and St Thomas' became more sharply distinguished and this led to medical students developing strong allegiances to a single institution through training and extra-curricular activities such as sports.[3]

The development of London Bridge Station in the 1860s led to St Thomas' relocating its hospital and medical school to a site adjacent to the Thames at the foot of Westminster Bridge, opposite the

Houses of Parliament. Queen Victoria laid the foundation stone on 13 May 1868 and formally opened the new hospital in 1871. Nurses had been employed throughout this period and Florence Nightingale established a nursing school at St Thomas' in 1860. Formal nurse training began at Guy's in 1877 with a Nurse Training School created three years later.[4] Guy's Dental School opened in 1888.[5] By the end of the nineteenth century, Guy's and St Thomas' were renowned teaching hospitals, and their expanding specialist areas supporting important medical discoveries attracted patients from across and beyond the UK.

The independence enjoyed by Guy's and St Thomas' enabled them to respond to the dramatic expansion in scientific knowledge, new practices, and technologies during the late nineteenth to early twentieth centuries. This led to the establishment of many new specialist departments, including orthopaedic surgery, psychiatry, thoracic surgery, diseases of children, dermatology, and neurology.[6] Hospital in-patient capacity increased through the creation of additional beds and the rising demand for out-patient services led to many innovations, such as the introduction of clinic booking systems. However, the financial impact of these developments was significant and the threat of 'impending bankruptcy' was a constant threat to the long-term security of both institutions through the 1920s and 1930s.[7] Financial pressures temporarily eased during the Second World War (1939–1945): although patients and staff were evacuated out of London, the hospitals remained open and received government money for providing casualty beds through the Emergency Medical Service (EMS).[8] These pressures returned when payments ceased after the war.[9] Annual expenditure at Guy's rose fourfold from £252,000 in 1938 to £900,000 in 1949, and the hospital only remained solvent through a £200,000 grant from the Ministry of Health.[10] At St Thomas', two-thirds of its 1947 total income of £626,000 came from government and local authority support.[11] Even more resources were now required to support the immediate post-war re-establishment of the hospitals and medical schools through short-term repairs and comprehensive rebuilding programmes. The nationalisation of the hospitals through the creation of a national health service provided a solution to these financial challenges.

The hospitals and the National Health Service (NHS)

Before and during the Second World War, concern about the need to improve healthcare across Britain led to a broad consensus around the concept of a national health service. The general expectation was that local authorities, already responsible for municipal hospitals and public health services such as vaccination and combatting infectious diseases, would oversee services within their localities. The anticipated trajectory of post-war health services was pushed off course by the unexpected landslide election victory of the Labour Party in 1945, which brought Clement Attlee's government into power and resulted in the appointment of Aneurin Bevan as Minister of Health responsible for creating a national service. Through three separate Acts for England and Wales, Scotland, and Northern Ireland, Bevan brought together existing voluntary and public services comprising over 3,000 hospitals, more than 415,000 staff members, 1,000s of GP practices, and a multitude of public health, dental, and eye services.[12] Alongside other teaching hospitals, Guy's and St Thomas' had feared that a nationalised system would compromise their independence and autonomy. In response to these concerns, Bevan agreed that teaching hospitals could report directly to the Ministry of Health rather than regional health authorities.[13]

Becoming part of the NHS on 5 July 1948 did not significantly alter the day-to-day working arrangements at Guy's and St Thomas'. The Boards of Governors retained supervision and the control of endowment funds, and direct lines of communication to the

Ministry of Health enabled the hospitals to remain autonomous. Rather, the change began to raise more fundamental questions about the very purpose of the hospitals and their relationship with local communities. Throughout their histories, development of the hospitals had been driven by the individual interests of medical staff and teaching requirements. They stood proud with international reputations for education and treatment. Now the hospitals became part of a group of neighbouring hospitals and over the following decades began to forge new ways of responding to local health needs.

Figure 1. The Hospital Groups in 1948 and 1960s

1948	
Guy's Hospital Group	**St Thomas' Hospital Group**
Guy's Hospital	St Thomas' Hospital
Nuffield House	St Thomas' Hospital Hydestile (wartime evacuation site)
York Clinic	St Thomas' Babies' Hostel
Evelina Hospital for Sick Children	Royal Waterloo Hospital for Women and Children
Eleanor Wemyss Home	General Lying-In Hospital
	Grosvenor Hospital for Women
	Roffey Park Rehabilitation Centre
Additions in 1960s	
St Olave's Hospital	Lambeth Group of Hospitals transferred to St Thomas' including Lambeth Hospital, Southwestern Hospital, Holmhurst
New Cross General Hospital	Southwestern Hospital
Dunoran Home	Roffey Park became an educational charity in 1967

Administration for a new era

During the 1950s, life in the hospitals and medical schools continued to be shaped by long-established, formal routines. Joachim Jose arrived in England on a boat from Portugal in 1955. Having served in the army, he had come to make a better life for himself at the age of 22. A friend working at St Thomas' arranged for him to visit the hospital's personnel office and, after the hospital had secured him a work permit from the Home Office, Joachim started work in the catering department in June 1956. This was the beginning of 42 years of service: 'I love this place. St Thomas' is part of my home. I don't know if I'm married to my wife or married to St Thomas'.' Morning routines began by setting up the Clerk to the Governors, Robert Pelham-Borley, for the day. The Clerk lived in a flat on the hospital site and after serving breakfast, including *The Times* newspaper, Joachim would polish the Clerk's shoes, brush his coat, and provide a red carnation for his buttonhole, purchased at the flower stall in Waterloo station. Joachim would then go to the dining room to finish serving breakfast to the doctors before cleaning the tables and setting out lunch: 'the doctors and consultants – they did like me very much and I did like them. From the beginning the doctors treated me like one of them, Jose can you do that for me? Jose, I have a meeting today, I need a [slide] carousel…I enjoyed every minute.'[14] Barbara Stevens joined St Thomas in 1962 as assistant cook, and in 1965 she secured a bursary funded by the hospital's endowment fund to train as a catering manager. At that time the hospital had its own butcher's shop and bakery and sourced all the vegetables from the local market. Barbara remembers the strong feeling of belonging to a family and noted that this was something that people working at Guy's would also have experienced at this time.

> People at Guy's would say the same. We were very privileged to be here when we were because the Clerk to the Governors, the Matron, they knew everybody right

down to the kitchen maid, the carpenter, the plumber and so forth. In my case I still have friends from literally 1962. You really had a feeling of family, and especially because so many of us in those days were resident as well. Just as the Clerk to the Governors was resident, so were the nurses, the physios, some of the cooks, the maids and so forth, so of course, there was an inclination to not only be working together but very often to socialise together as well.[15]

There were many instances of staff finding future partners through work. Luis Ribeiro, a fellow Portuguese, began working in the doctors' dining room in 1969, fell in love and married Krystyna who had come from Poland to work in the catering department and stayed at the hospital until retiring in 2004.[16]

Following Robert Pelham-Borley's retirement in 1962, a new era for St Thomas' was ushered in with the appointment of Bryan McSwiney as the new Clerk to the Governors. Bryan had been a trainee administrator at St Thomas' and his father, Professor B A McSwiney, served as Dean of the Medical School from 1940 to 1947. Bryan joined St Thomas' in September 1948 and spent the first year attached to different departments. He remembered that 'each ward had a kitchen equipped with a solid fuel AGA on which the nurses made tea for the patients and boiled eggs for those who were fortunate to have eggs brought in by relatives'. Food was rationed up to 1955 and building permits had to be obtained for any building work: 'the windows of the hospital were still covered with netting glued to the glass to prevent injury from shattered glass'.[17] In 1962 Bryan returned to St Thomas' as Clerk to the Governors and over the next 12 years, his vision and determination drove the institution's development and its adoption of new responsibilities for the health of local communities. Bryan's response to the Ministry of Health's 10-Year Plan for the Development of Hospitals in England and Wales was to propose St Thomas' provide more services for the local population in Lambeth.[18] Prior to the establishment of the NHS, Lambeth Hospital had been one of the largest municipal hospitals and became part of the Lambeth Hospital Group in 1948. A working party of governors and the Lambeth Hospital Group management committee agreed that, rather than dividing provision between the two hospitals, they should be amalgamated with the eventual transfer of Lambeth Hospital services to the St Thomas' site. These changes coincided with a proposal that medical student numbers be increased, which in turn would require a greater number of hospital beds to support clinical training. The outcome was an agreement that St Thomas' would provide 'hospital facilities as are required by a population of some 200,000 persons residing in and around North Lambeth'. This would entail the provision of 1,255 beds.[19]

Bryan recognised that bringing Lambeth into St Thomas' called for new thinking about health needs at a local population level. Together with Bob Nevin, Dean of the Medical School, Bryan approached Walter Holland, an alumnus of St Thomas' who had returned from a fellowship in epidemiology at Johns Hopkins University in the US. 'The fundamental question of what and how much care should/ could be provided was the subject of an intense debate in which I participated,' recounted Walter.[20] The cost of such investigative work was considerable, and Bryan and Walter agreed that an application be made to the Ministry of Health to create a Health Services Research Unit underwritten by St Thomas' endowment fund. This enabled work to proceed immediately, and the application was approved in due course. St Thomas' Social Medicine and Health Services Research Unit became the first of its kind in the UK. It had both a research and teaching function and was distinctive for its multidisciplinary team, including epidemiologists, economists, sociologists, and medical statisticians. Walter also established connections to the London School of Economics' Department of Social Administration.[21] The Lambeth studies revealed that services for disabled people, community care, and general practice all required attention. One outcome was the creation of a committee of community medicine, bringing together St Thomas', general practices, and local authority services to address gaps in provision.

The amalgamation of Lambeth with St Thomas' transformed the rebuilding programme established to address the ravages of war. In June 1963, architects Yorke Rosenberg Mardall were instructed that the new scheme should 'allow for the maximum flexibility in the future having regard to the requirements of medical teaching, to possible changes in population and catchment area, and to the effect of the redevelopment of hospital services in neighbouring areas'.[22] They presented their proposals in January 1964 and although plans for Phase 1 (East Wing) were unchanged, Phases 2 and 3 had undergone 'drastic revision' to take account of planning requirements about overall building height and the increase in bed numbers.[23] The East Wing opened in 1966 with 196 beds, operating theatres, outpatient departments, and laboratories.[24] The new building symbolised the reconfiguration of St Thomas' within local health services: as Treasurer and Chairman of the Governors, John Prideaux, noted in 1966, 'assuming a dual role as a teaching hospital and a district hospital [is] something that would have been regarded as impracticable a few years ago...[it is now] designed to care for a local population in terms of present-day human need'.[25]

Over his tenure, Bryan instigated a culture of professional aspiration across his administrative team. He developed close relationships between administrators and medical staff, and was the first clerk invited to attend meetings of the medical and surgical officers; Bryan was even given the privilege of using their dining room. These developments were important in establishing administration as an equal of medicine, and practically beneficial, providing opportunities for the informal exchange of opinions.[26] He introduced a nightly rota so that any complaints, security incidents, or other crises could be dealt with by an administrative duty officer, rather than adding to the work of medical and nursing staff.[27] Bryan built his leadership team through recruiting trainees from the NHS Administrators' Training Scheme, run by the King's Fund in London and the University of Manchester's Department of Public Administration.[28] In 1965, he set up a Development and Research Team (DART), which became the subject of much interest from other hospital authorities. The creation of the NHS had raised questions about how to create 'new kinds of skill' in health service administration.[29] Now DART began to undertake problem-solving on a project basis, enabling new approaches to be brought to bear on the increasing complexity of this domain.

The 1968 winter flu epidemic caused 'chaos' at St Thomas' with a huge increase in patient admissions. Richard Sawyer, who had joined as Planning Assistant and Deputy Hospital Secretary in 1966, was tasked with creating an admissions system. St Thomas' had around 500 beds at that point and the consultants 'owned' the beds in the wards they managed. There was no limit on the number of beds per ward: 'on every one of those Nightingale wards they'd just fill every space within, even the entrance corridors...which did nobody any good because then normal beds for admission were blocked'. Richard began by speaking to each consultant to analyse bed requirements per ward. Then, sitting in his workroom in the basement, he worked out a system on a large board covered with magnetic pieces representing wards and beds. Each bed included the patient's name, date of admission, and anticipated discharge. When complete, the board was transferred into 'an admissions place where everybody could go and see which beds were physically free, and who was responsible for them'. Richard's achievement in getting consultants to agree to work within their bed allocation and not encroach on other wards was huge given the supremacy of clinicians at that time. It illustrates Bryan's success in establishing administration as an important dimension of clinical work. The project also led to the appointment of a fulltime admissions officer in 1969, trained by Richard and his colleagues. The acceptance of this role across the hospitals made Richard 'very pleased'.[30]

While not lavish with praise, Bryan picked people who 'made things happen' and imbued them with a 'can-do attitude'. Many of his trainees enjoyed long and influential careers in health services. One former trainee noted that working with Bryan gave them the confidence to stand 'side by side with [medical staff] and say, we are professional too. In the way that you may do your medicine or surgery, we will be aspiring to do exactly the same in our administrator role'.[31] The fact that some of Bryan's trainees were instrumental in setting up the Guy's and St Thomas' research project, the output of which is this book, speaks to the legacy of his contribution to the institution and its people.

Building for a new era

'Get on, or Get out' was the motto at Guy's in the 1950s, expressing the institution's ambition to produce 'academic leaders of the profession…first-class family doctors and dental surgeons'.[32] Yet the war-damaged buildings within which care and teaching took place still left much to be desired. Sandra Carnall Ferrelly's lasting memory of her visit to Guy's as a 14-year-old patient was the squalid nature of the clinic, in which consultants' desks were positioned in each corner of a room, and the lack of screens or curtains made private conversations impossible. After leaving school, Sandra attended a business administration secretarial course and in the summer of 1962 was invited to interviews at Guy's and St Thomas' on the same day. After half an hour of her morning interview at St Thomas', 'it transpired they thought I was coming to be interviewed for a nurse and told me not to waste their time'. In the afternoon she had a highly formal interview at Guy's for a position as junior assistant on commissioning of the New Guy's House. Sandra began work on 13 August and continued working at Guy's for more than 30 years. She had 'wonderful' support from John Carruthers, who oversaw the non-clinical support departments and building development, and Lady Boland, interior designer and wife of the Dean of the Medical

School, Rowan Boland: 'they realised I had a brain and so they got me education'. Guy's financed her training in interior design at the Hammersmith College of Art and then supported her to gain a Higher National Certificate in structural engineering and building.

As Sandra has observed, Guy's vision that interior design was a critical part of the rebuilding programme was radical: 'I don't know at that time there were any other people doing it'. This approach produced a synergy between the design and function of spaces that directly benefited patients and staff. To fit out the new wards, Lady Boland worked with various domestic companies – including Parker Knoll – to design furniture, including bedside lockers and wardrobes. Much of the hospital furniture used today originated from this initiative. The nurses' accommodation was designed as 'something that was effectively a ship's cabin, so not an inch of space was wasted, and everything was built in'.

However, the patriarchal culture proved challenging for Sandra. Within a few months of starting work, one of the senior surgeons pushed her against the side of the lift in New Guy's House and put his hand up her skirt. Having complained to her colleagues, she was summoned to see the governors and 'told that it was not up to me to make a fuss about things, the senior surgeons were senior surgeons and had to be treated with respect, and if I didn't like it, there's the door'. On Lady Boland's retirement, Sandra applied for her job but was turned down on account of being female; the fact she might marry and have children was viewed as a major disadvantage. However, the male appointee did not stay long and the arrival of a new personnel officer who challenged embedded views about female employees resulted in Sandra's appointment to the role. Despite loving the work, she soon realised interior design was generally dismissed as trivial by 'the male-dominated architect building community', a matter of paint colours rather than an intrinsic part of the design and build of hospital spaces. After some lobbying, Guy's created a specific role for her as development works administrator.

During the 1960s, Guy's acquired additional hospitals including St Olave's Hospital, New Cross Hospital, and Dunoran House. Sandra's first independent project was to redesign a house to accommodate nurses working in the adjacent Dunoran House. Originally a convalescent home set up by Dr Barbara Morton of the Bermondsey Medical Mission, Dunoran had developed into a nursing facility for patients with terminal cancer or neurological disorders.[33] Another early job was the upgrade of the ante- and post-natal clinic, situated in the out-patient extension to Hunt's House. A large, scrubbed pine table sat in the middle of the clinic. One end was used to test patient urine samples; the other supported an extremely large paper sack of Ostermilk for making up babies' bottles. The slope on the table meant any spilt urine would trickle down towards the paper sack. When Sandra told the clinic nurses the table must be removed, they said, 'Oh, we've always had that table' and complained to Matron. Matron overruled their protest, and the table was removed. Designing new spaces from scratch required Sandra to develop a deep understanding of space and function. When planning the new mortuary, she spent a lot of time watching staff carry out the various processes. Concerned she was missing something, Sandra asked the technician to talk her through each specific stage from first receiving a body. It was only through doing this that she discovered they used a bucket to rinse down the rubber sheets. Thus, at the last moment, the design was changed to include a large sink. Sandra kept the patient's view at the forefront: 'I was able to say, when you're in the ward, these are the things that matter. Not the obvious kind of things that men, particularly young architects, notice. But things about being kept awake all night because the kitchen where the nurses go for tea and a chat is opposite your bed and the door clanks and bangs.' For Sandra, this innovative approach reflected the broader spirit of Guy's, which empowered its staff to engage with change and challenge the

21

status quo: 'We were the naughty boys who wanted to change the world. Whereas St Thomas' were the prefects.'[34]

Medical education in London

The hospitals and their respective medical schools had always enjoyed a symbiotic relationship, with the hospitals supporting the development of students' clinical skills, and students providing hands-on care for patients. In 1910, Abraham Flexner's report on medical education recommending that students be trained within a university setting to sustain better linkages with the sciences and other disciplines, set the agenda for much of twentieth-century medical education development across Europe and North America.[35] The first significant move to address this in the UK came in 1942. Sir William Goodenough, deputy chairman of Barclays Bank and co-founder of the Nuffield Provincial Hospitals Trust, led an enquiry into the organisation and distribution of medical schools, arrangements for teaching staff, and the provision of science and clinical teaching facilities. The focus was on the particular problems of London: the clustering of many small medical schools in central London at a time when the local population was decreasing had led to insufficient clinical training material for students. The resulting 1944 report positioned medical education as the 'essential foundation' of the anticipated comprehensive health service, recommended that all medical schools be linked to a university, and proposed that medical education become less vocational and include more science-based teaching.[36] Child health, psychiatry, and social medicine were identified for development, and payments to medical schools were to be withheld if an appropriate proportion of women were not recruited as medical students.[37] To address the issue in London, the report suggested linking municipal hospitals to specific medical schools, and that acute hospital services be developed beyond central London by relocating St George's, Charing Cross, and the Royal Free hospitals to the peripheries.

In 1968, a Royal Commission on Medical Education chaired by Lord Todd recommended reducing the overall number of medical schools in London through pairing: Guy's with King's College Hospital Medical School, and St Thomas' with St George's Hospital Medical School.[38] The institutions protested vociferously against the proposals. Notably, the focus of concerns was not so much on the philosophical question of becoming attached to a university but about the loss of identity that mergers would generate for individual medical schools. The Commission also recommended setting up a London medical education committee with an independent chairman and members and representatives from the University Grants Committee, the University of London, and the Department of Health and Social Security. This was initially rejected by the University of London and a working party was not constituted until 1971. In 1974, it was announced that the proposals relating to Guy's and St Thomas' medical schools would be set aside for five years due to high site costs and the time it would take to implement transitions.

Student experiences

At this point the medical curriculum was consistent across most UK medical schools. While the first year's *Medicinae Baccalaureus* (MB) course covered chemistry, zoology, and botany, most students had studied sciences at school and entered directly into the second year MB course, focused on non-clinical training including dissection, physiology, biochemistry, and related subjects. The last three years at medical school centred on clinical training for the final MB.

Family connections often took precedence over educational achievement for gaining a place at medical school. When Jan Organe failed her physics A-level in 1958, her father telephoned the Dean of St Thomas' Medical School, Bob Nevin: 'no problem', was the immediate response, 'she can do first MB' next year.[39] Dundas Moore left school with no A-levels, but once he had completed national service, his father – a Guy's alumnus – arranged an interview and he was allocated a place at Guy's in 1958: 'This is frowned upon nowadays, but I think if you look back, in retrospect, I don't think we've done too badly.' Family connections stretched over generations. According to Dundas, a popular saying among nurses was that you 'went to the London Hospital to learn to be a nurse, you went to St Thomas' Hospital to learn to be a lady, and you went to Guy's Hospital to find a husband. And as my mother met my father, my sister met her husband and I met my wife at Guy's, I suppose I couldn't really argue against it.'[40] Richard Hughes trained at Guy's in the early 1960s, the third generation of his family to do so. His grandmother and mother were Guy's nurses and his cousins trained there and married Guy's alumni: 'I doubt whether there's any other family which has quite so many members attached to Guy's Hospital. I think there was a sort of tacit assumption that Guy's was the place you had to go to. There was never ever any thought that I would go anywhere else.'[41]

Students without connections to the medical school or medicine in general found it harder though Guy's and St Thomas' were natural and prestigious destinations for Oxbridge students. The struggle to establish high-quality clinical training in Oxford and Cambridge led to a pattern of elite students attending Oxbridge for pre-clinical studies and then transferring to London medical schools for clinical training that endured well into the 1970s.[42] 'I nearly didn't get in,' said Cyril Chantler, who undertook his pre-clinical training at Cambridge and was advised by his tutor that Guy's 'was a good place'.

> I was interviewed by a group of gentlemen, all exactly the same and they started off the conversation by saying was my father a Guy's man? I said, no, he wasn't a Guy's man and they said, but he is a doctor? And I said, no, he's not a doctor and then somebody else said, well, do you have any connection with the medical profession? And I said, my grandfather was a pharmacist and had a chemist shop in

Bury in Lancashire where I come from and my mother's a pharmacist and they said, anything else? I said, no, and there was silence and then I said, oh, yes, I said, my sister's a nurse in St Thomas'. So, they said, well, why don't you go to St Thomas'? I said, because she recommended Guy's and that got me in, I think![43]

The stereotype of a typical Guy's or St Thomas' medical student being a White Anglo-Saxon Protestant male certainly seems to hold true for this period. Guy's and St Thomas' had been two of seven London medical schools that refused to admit women during the First World War.[44] By the 1930s, Guy's offered a limited number of places to women on their postgraduate courses and was willing to admit some female MB students by 1944.[45] But change happened very slowly. When Penny Hewitt applied to Guy's in 1956 the interview panel included one female doctor from London County Council; at that time, Guy's had no female consultants. Penny was among 20 female students admitted in a cohort of 100 students, the highest ratio of female to male students in Guy's history. Penny's older brother had trained at Guy's, and she found it to be a very close-knit community: 'There was a wonderful medical school secretary called Arthur Wallace who seemed to know everything about everybody. He would see my father walking in, and he would immediately tell him about what my brother was doing and what I was doing. Incredible chap.' She does not remember sensing any resistance to female students, but the culture of the institution was male-oriented and placed great emphasis on sports such as rugby. When attempting to join the Golf Society on Freshers' Day, Penny was told 'it's men only'.[46] This rebuttal led her to form a women's golfing society; the sport would later become a mixed activity at Guy's. In 1960, the cohort of medical students admitted to St Thomas' comprised 43 male and eight female students. A single student came from overseas and only two students had not been educated in public schools.[47]

Lifelong friendships were established during training. 'I remember St Thomas's with great affection: I have never met so many talented people devoted to making lives better, not with any sanctimony but almost continuous, unassuming humour. My first day in the student bar I was delighted to see pints of Scotch Ale being passed through the open window to someone hanging upside down to improve his potholing powers,' noted Alexander Macdonald.[48] Dissection provided an early bonding experience. This was studied in small groups and accounted for around 700 hours of curriculum time. 'You got to be a very close team with the people you were actually doing the dissection with. You knew who was good, head down, getting on with the job and who was the chap with all the book knowledge, and who turned up, and who was punctual, and you got a good working relationship with your contemporaries,' said Penny Hewitt about Guy's. When Peter Christie entered St Thomas' in 1958, the Professor of Anatomy was Dai Davies, who had joined the School in 1948 and was then editor of *Gray's Anatomy*, the world-renowned anatomical textbook. Peter remembers sitting in the old-fashioned lecture theatre with his fellow students and being told by Dai that 'you have to learn *Gray's* off by heart'. Peter's cohort included a small group of women, 'all absolutely brilliant girls'. However, during the first session Dai cautioned the women: 'Don't forget', he said, 'that St Thomas' Hospital was the last medical school to allow women in.' Peter remembers the girls 'disappearing below their desks, trying not to be seen'.[49] Women students may have been small in number, but these early cohorts provided their male counterparts with strong competition. Hywel Thomas had qualified as a biochemist at the University of Wales in Cardiff and joined St Thomas' department of biochemistry in 1968. He remembers the female students, though few in number, as 'exceedingly bright and very, very well-qualified, very intellectual and very, very sharp, so some of the boys then had quite a job keeping up with their women compatriots'.[50]

Teaching at both schools reflected the style of the times and was mainly lecture-based with some tutorials and assessment through examination. At Guy's, Tim Clark found plenty of time to play cricket: 'the summer term, when we dissected the abdomen thorax, I never went in because I was playing cricket all the time. So, there wasn't tremendous pressure to study…It was not like today where lectures have to have objectives, you have to hand in the coursework. It was very much you toddled along to a lecture if you felt like it. The lecturer gave his lecture using a blackboard. That was it. Then you had to read your books yourself. It was quite different from today. But I liked it'.[51] Alan Maryon Davis remembers St Thomas' as 'very old-fashioned' during that period: 'it was a bit of a backward institution in those days, a bit of it died in the war and it had to be, kind of, almost dragged into the twentieth century. I'm glad to say things have changed a lot now and I have to say that, because I'm still employed by them!'.[52] The style of teaching meant that 'some students, who perhaps weren't so confident could easily be humiliated, it wasn't a good way of teaching. I think that anybody that was taught in that era would recognise that,' reflected Tina Challacombe, who studied at Guy's during the 1950s.[53] Despite the flaws, meeting teachers who were conducting pioneering research could be life-transforming. As a student, Ian Cameron fell into conversation with Stephen Semple, Professor of Medicine at St Thomas', whose work on respiration was charting new territory.[54] That encounter 'was the beginning of my career in trying to elucidate how respiration was controlled'.[55]

Despite the formality of relationships, social mixing between students, hospital, and medical school staff was an important part of life. The bar at St Thomas' was a hub for 'stimulating conversation,' recalls David Barlow, who trained during the 1960s: 'There was no side there. You got there and the Professor of Medicine would be there, a porter would be there, a second-year medical student would be there. And anybody could talk to anybody. Sharpey-Schafer [Professor of Medicine] was the one who actually…instituted the rule that everybody should buy their own drinks because otherwise you'd have the whole team there and the junior doctor would end up spending much more than they could afford buying a round for everybody, so we had this rule, we always bought our own drinks. That was the setting of an important part of my life.'[56] Guy's could also be a 'very friendly, relaxed place' outside of formal teaching: 'if you were a medical student and you met a consultant walking across the park or something, you know, he'd talk to you. It wasn't a sort of them and us, which existed a lot in London hospitals in the 1950s and 1960s'.[57]

Entering the wards

Between ten and 20 per cent of students undertook their two-year pre-clinical training at Oxford or Cambridge before joining the medical schools for clinical experience. Cyril Chantler found his clinical training at Guy's to be a match made in heaven: 'I realised that my life's choice was correct the day I walked into Guy's as a clinical student in 1960, I thought, oh, this is just wonderful! I mean, I can't think of anything better than being a doctor and I'm being constantly surprised that anybody pays me to do what, in fact, is not just my work, but my hobby. I think it's just a fantastic privilege to be a doctor and Guy's was a fantastic place to learn it, because the staff there were tremendously devoted to the students.' Nevertheless, relationships between students and consultants were not always cosy.

> Some of the consultants were a bit off-putting and they didn't always perhaps interact with patients in quite the way I thought doctors and patients should interact. But then I went, in my second clinical year, to study paediatrics and I thought the paediatricians were just fantastic! They seemed much more, to me, like doctors ought to be. People like, Philip Evans who I succeeded at Guy's and Ronald McKeith who was an extraordinary, charismatic, wonderful man who more or less invented developmental paediatrics himself throughout the world. These were the

28

sort of people you met, so I can't imagine anything better than having been a doctor and having been at Guy's'. [58]

Like Cyril, Alan Maryon Davis had done his pre-clinical training at Cambridge. Before leaving school, he read widely about the human body and its physiology but had also been inspired to enter medicine by the 1954 British comedy film, *Doctor in the House,* based on Richard Gordon's 1952 novel. This charted the adventures of a group of students through medical school and featured a bombastic senior surgeon, Sir Lancelot Spratt. Arriving at St Thomas' in 1965, Alan was immediately struck by 'the horrific hierarchy' and the 'god-like' groups of consultants and senior nursing staff.

> The consultants were still, in those days, quite God-like, you know, a bit like Sir Lancelot Spratt. They still had the waistcoats and the gold chains and the half glasses, and all that sort of stuff, and they still treated lower people very badly. The other sort of God-like people were the matrons and the sisters, they were the ones who had to be obeyed and even the consultants trod very carefully around the senior nursing staff. So, first impressions were of these hierarchies and how we medical students had to kowtow an awful lot and fit in very carefully to the shark-infested waters that we were entering into. [59]

Clinical teaching was undertaken on an apprenticeship basis. Small groups of students were allocated to a medical or surgical 'firm', each headed by two or three consultants supported by a team of junior medical staff. As medical students we 'were really very heavily involved with their patients,' remembered Richard Hughes.

> You felt you were involved with the care of the patients. You saw your patient every day. When they came in you would do a blood count on them; you would test their

urine and record the results in the notes…The junior medical students learnt from the senior medical students; we all learnt from the registrars and the consultants…some of the patients became very attached to us and appreciative of what we did for them. We would wheel them along to the theatres, we would be in the theatres throughout the operations, we would go back with them.[60]

Students were given responsibility for a small number of patients and, as Tina Challacombe has described, 'expected to be rigorously asked questions by the consultant and/or registrar' during the regular ward rounds: 'That gave us a lot of impetus to find out about the illness that that patient had, because you didn't want to be made to look as if you didn't know about the case.'[61]

Medical and surgical firms were on a rota for emergency admissions with the on-call firm living in the hospital for a week. The accommodation included a common room and kitchen, and the firm's students were expected to prepare a meal every night: 'That was a great activity, a great feature of student life. Even people who were undomesticated would learn to cook as a student when they were on the surgical firm. One night during the week they'd invite all the medical people as guests. You were given £10 by the medical school to feed all these people in this midnight feast that we'd have fitting around emergencies. The better meal you could produce, and the better entertainment you could lay on, the more your status of being a good firm rose.'[62] The long working hours created opportunities for learning and camaraderie as students and staff discussed the difficult cases that they were dealing with on that take.

One of the radical changes at St Thomas' in the early 1960s was the introduction of bleeps, invented by Peter Styles in the physical medicine department. This enabled the anaesthetic department to introduce the 'Crash Call System' so that anaesthetists could be directed to emergencies as quickly as possible. 'It was marvellous', according to Jean Davenport, a secretary, although on one occasion an anaesthetist was so annoyed to be called during his lunch 'that he dunked his bleep in the water jug'.[63]

The expectation that each hospital would be staffed by its alumni was so strong that the St Thomas' application form was not designed for outside entrants. Barry Jackson trained at Westminster Medical School and carried out house officer jobs on the Westminster 'circuit'. He applied to St Thomas' Hospital for a junior appointment in cardiac surgery.

> I was so appalled by the structure of the form that I very nearly didn't apply because it was clearly directed only at St Thomas' graduates. There were such questions as what, if any, prizes did you win in the medical school, and such like. Which of our several sporting clubs were you associated with? There was no space for referees, but rather you had to put a passport photograph of yourself at the top right-hand corner so they could recognise you.

Barry telephoned the medical staffing office and was advised to write the name of two referees on the back of the form. In the event he was appointed without interview and subsequently discovered that St Thomas' had not contacted his named referees but instead discussed his application with a different clinician: 'That couldn't happen today.'[64]

Nursing and midwifery

Nurses formed equally deep attachments to their training institutions. The Nurses' League at Guy's had been formed in 1900 by Matron Sarah Swift.[65] By the 1950s, the League incorporated a wide range of extracurricular activities, such as the Nurses' Choral Society, and maintained strong links with Guy's alumni. The solid hierarchies and daily routines that had shaped nursing since its professionalisation continued through the post-war period, with students subject to strict timetables and schedules from their first day. The average working week could be around 52 hours and opportunities for socialisation outside the Nurses' Home were limited; student nurses would spend Saturday mornings cleaning the Chapel.[66] At St Thomas', Grace Jones began her midwifery training in 1952. This involved spending six months in a hospital and six months in the community. Grace struggled to sleep during her first few nights in the nurses' home on the corner of Westminster Bridge due to the chimes of Big Ben. It was usual at that time for new mothers to spend up to two weeks on the ward recovering, largely confined to their beds. 'Babies were labelled in the nursery so we could identify them and there was virtually no security on the wards. The smog in London was so bad that in the early 1950s some of the babies had dirt around their noses.'[67]

Kay Riley also studied nursing at St Thomas' in 1949. After training in midwifery and working in Canada she returned as a ward sister and remained at the institution for the rest of her working life. The strong community spirit enhanced the work: 'you knew personally the carpenters, and the plumbers, and the engineers, and the domestic supervisors who worked in your wards so that when you were wanting things you knew the carpenter intimately, and he knew exactly what you wanted, and he would come very promptly and see to things. You didn't have to write out in those days a request form and say why you needed something. You just rang him up and he came'.

Daily ward routines were topped and tailed by morning and evening prayers read by the ward sister.

> She came in as Big Ben struck eight o'clock exactly, not a minute early or late, and she knelt at the desk in the centre

of the ward with her nurses all around her on their knees and had these set prayers. They were brief. About three minutes. And then in the evening the same thing happened at eight o'clock at night. Regardless of what was going on in the ward, anybody such as consultants, registrars, doctors visiting in the ward automatically knew these were taking place so they would carry on with their work, or just be quiet, but they knew they were taking place. They were very much appreciated by the patients who often commented on them.

Beyond the wards, the Chapel was 'the centre of the hospital' and offered Sunday services, including an early service for staff before they went on duty; a morning service to which patients would be wheeled down in their beds or in wheelchairs to attend; and a Roman Catholic service in the afternoon. Each Saturday the chaplain would visit the wards to find patients who would like to take communion on Sunday. Kay remembers one 'lovely old Lambethian lady' being asked if she would like Holy Communion: 'she replied, what is that? If it's free and on the National Health, then I'll have it'. Ward sisters would also hold services in sitting rooms where there was a piano, with hymns, readings, and prayers that were 'very much appreciated by the patients'. The opening of the East Wing in 1966 made it harder for nurses to maintain these religious practices as the wards were designed as four-bedded bays. This meant patients could not easily hear the prayers being said. Kay circumvented the problem by installing a microphone and continued the practice of daily prayers through to her retirement in 1987. [68] Caroline Cave began nurse training in 1973 and her set was the first to wear paper caps because of difficulties sourcing lace for the frilly caps. She remembered the daily routine of prayers, 'patients of all faiths, or no faiths, seemed to like the practice'.[69]

Deborah Hofman remembers the pride taken in everyday practices such as giving patients a bed bath. She began nurse training at St Thomas' in 1969 and described the sister on City ward as 'a dragon'. But when Deborah herself became ill, she was admitted to City ward and nursed by the sister herself.

> I had a very, very high temperature and immediately a jug of iced fresh-squeezed lemon juice was put on my table, and I was put in a corner bed, so very quiet. I just felt in a completely safe pair of hands. I knew what was going to happen and when it was going to happen. You could just lie back and relax, as it were.[70]

Excellent nursing care was integral to some of the new medical technologies of the time, such as dialysis. At the age of 20, Francis Tibbles spent many weeks at St Thomas' undergoing dialysis before he was able to transfer to home treatment.

> When I was an inpatient [the nursing staff on the wards] were really fantastic and so friendly. I think they had more time in those days, because they literally sometimes would sit by your bed for five or six minutes and speak to you...I just found all the nurses, and also some of the housemen as well who were in [the consultant] team, they were always very interested, would ask any questions, would give you time if you needed that time to ask them things. I never felt any short temperedness or keenness to get away. They seemed to have a lot of patience with me when I needed that.[71]

Nurses also enjoyed high standing in the local community and Betsy Morley who trained at Guy's in the 1950s remembered being given free fruit from Borough Market, 'for the Bermondsey people, Guy's nurses...could do no wrong which was a marvellous feeling'.[72]

Communities and rivalries

Daily life at Guy's and St Thomas' was shaped by a strong sense of community and for patients, staff, and students, each institution operated as a family. Bonds were built through events that brought everyone together to celebrate special occasions and times of the year. Every Christmas at St Thomas', as Kay Riley reflected, 'we had a very authentic nativity play that was organised by one of the sisters. Rehearsals took place for weeks beforehand...the play was done to absolute perfection, using a new-born baby from the midwifery unit...[the sister] was so particular with getting perfect gowns and costumes that we weren't even allowed to sit down in case the garments got creased before the play started. It ran for four nights, and the Chapel was always full, every night'.[73]

Sport was also an integral part of institutional life and medical school interviews were used as an opportunity to identify future sporting talent. Alan Maryon Davis had been interviewed by a group of 'furious-looking senior doctors' who asked him which sports he played. 'I had to confess I wasn't much of a sports person really,' said Alan, 'I said, I do ballroom dancing and bellringing and they looked at each other, askance!'[74] When Stephen Challacombe arrived at Guy's to study dentistry in 1964 he was surprised at the high standards of play: 'Slightly to my horror, when we arrived here, the hospital ran ten rugby sides a week and it took me a couple of years to get into the first 15 and my career subsequently was, as a student, a very nice mixture of playing rugby three times a week, playing water polo twice a week and doing research for one afternoon a week...that's really the pattern of my life subsequently, of sport, hard work and research, so it's been a very good mix.'[75]

Despite the apparent similarities between the institutions there were deep cultural differences.

Guy's in its heyday, I would say, apart from the fact that it was a very relaxed and friendly place to work, it wasn't the least bit hierarchical…it was entrepreneurial in a way that, for instance, Thomas' never was. And that was a major difference. St Thomas', as I see it, reckoned to be a very good district general hospital; to provide an excellent casualty service and an excellent service to its local community. But it wasn't the least bit entrepreneurial. It didn't establish, you know, new developments in medicine.[76]

Positioned across from the Houses of Parliament, St Thomas' was perceived as 'upper-class', with strong connections to political and social networks of power. Guy's maintained the feel of a local hospital. The community was protective towards students and staff, and students visiting the Old King's Head pub in Borough High Street would be treated to drinks by locals.

We were also very fond of our local borough community, which were very much part of the ethos of the hospital, that we looked after them and they looked after us. In the 1950s a female on their own didn't tend to walk round the back streets of London on their own at night time, but if you walked round the London borough of Southwark with your Guy's scarf on you felt safe because people were, 'Oh, you know, you looked after Granny when she was ill, we'll look after you and make sure you're all right'. There was a very nice sort of local supportive atmosphere … One wouldn't have done it in the back streets anywhere in London, but round Guy's as a Guy's person with your Guy's things on you were okay. [77]

The rivalry between Guy's and St Thomas' came into its own in the sports arena. St Thomas' was Guy's strongest competitor and the longer history of the institutions shaped and stoked this adversarial relationship. 'I knew that Thomas Guy was a governor of St Thomas' and that Guy's was an offshoot. But there was just a general feeling that it was like family rivalry. They were the big brother that you always rebelled against. And also, there was the feeling that Thomas' was rather a posh place, and they thought Guy's was in trade, and we were the grammar schoolboys, and they were the public schoolboys. I'm sure that's not true, but that was the nature of the rivalry,' reflected Tim Clark.[78] From a St Thomas' perspective, Alan Maryon Davis remembers the 'blood-curdling rivalry' of his student days around sporting activities: 'they were at each other's throats, constantly stealing each other's mascots and sticking them up in some far-flung place, you know, or dragging them through the streets! No, it was an intense rivalry'.[79]

Conclusion

The first decades of the NHS were transformative for Guy's and St Thomas', with major rebuilding programmes, the development of new services and ways of working, and most significantly, a shift towards hospitals taking on responsibility for meeting the health needs of their local populations. In many respects the new NHS was beneficial for the institutions as it provided long-term financial security whilst allowing them much freedom and autonomy in the governance and development of the hospitals. Things were to change significantly in 1974 with the first structural reorganisation of the NHS.

CHAPTER THREE

From Hospitals to Caring for Local Communities, 1970-1979

Overview

The 1970s proved to be a turbulent decade for Guy's and St Thomas'. The first NHS structural reorganisation in 1974 broke historical patterns of governance by removing the Boards of Governors and establishing direct accountability to the new Lambeth, Southwark, and Lewisham Area Health Authority (AHA) (Teaching). Whereas Guy's and St Thomas' had benefited from increasing financial resources through the 1950s and 1960s with good access to capital funding supported by endowment funds, they now found themselves to be in the eye of the storm. Britain was badly affected by the global oil crisis and by 1976 the Labour Government had to apply to the International Monetary Fund for a loan. This led to deep cuts in public expenditure and the Government sought to control inflation by holding down pay levels. The fall in real wages led to industrial strike action across the NHS. Guy's and St Thomas' suffered heavy reductions in budgets through the introduction of a new formula for distributing funding across the NHS and by the end of the decade, the Government appointed commissioners to take over the Lambeth, Southwark, and Lewisham AHA's responsibilities as they refused to work within the defined budget cash limits although this decision was later challenged and overturned.

Hospital groups to districts

The 1973 National Health Service Reorganisation Act which was implemented from 1 April 1974 marked a decisive point in the history of Guy's and St Thomas'. The coming of the NHS in 1948 had brought financial relief to the institutions and although they were encouraged to engage more directly with the needs of their local communities, the historical patterns of governance through the Boards of Governors continued. The institutions retained control over their endowment funds which gave them the financial wherewithal to support and develop activities in line with institutional frameworks of vision and purpose. Little opposition was encountered from the Ministry of Health and as the previous chapter showed, the excellent political networks enjoyed by St Thomas' in particular, had enabled close relationships with ministers and civil servants that led to the successful acquisition of capital funding. The 1974 reorganisation disrupted these ways of working and posed a significant threat to the autonomy of the institutions.

The 1974 reorganisation created Area Health Authorities (AHAs) which were overseen by the top management tier of Regional Health Authorities (RHAs). AHAs had responsibility for providing comprehensive healthcare for a given population living in a defined geographical area and were divided into Districts which took on new responsibilities for community health services as these had previously been under the authority of local councils. Teaching hospitals including Guy's and St Thomas', which had previously reported directly to the Ministry of Health, were placed under control of AHAs, and local District Management Teams (DMTs) assumed oversight of hospital and community health services across each District. The Boards of Governors were dissolved although the introduction of Special Trustees enabled the institutions to maintain control of endowment funds.

The South East Thames RHA had oversight of five new AHAs including the Lambeth, Lewisham, and Southwark AHA (Teaching) which assumed responsibility for the Guy's and St Thomas' Hospital Groups. Four new health districts were created: Guy's, St Thomas', King's and Lewisham. Guy's Health District included the Evelina Hospital for Sick Children, the Royal Dental, Saint Olave's and New Cross Hospitals; St Thomas' Health District included the Grosvenor Hospital for Women, Lambeth, Royal Eye, Royal Waterloo, South Western and Tooting Bec Hospitals.[1] St Thomas', which had been within the South West Thames RHA, was moved to the South East Thames RHA, producing much discontent across the institution.[2] The shift also altered longstanding patterns around the rotation of junior medical staff and patient flows.

Many personnel across Guy's and St Thomas' took advantage of the plethora of new administrative and finance posts that had been created in RHAs and AHAs and applied for promotion. In 1948, staff holding senior positions such as the clerk of the governors and the chief nursing officer were automatically transferred to the equivalent roles within the institution. But times had changed and appointments to the new health district were through a formal and open application process. Two of the key figures at St Thomas', Bryan McSwiney, Clerk of the Governors, and Sheila Garrett, Chief Nursing Officer, decided not to seek reappointment. Bryan McSwiney retained his connection with St Thomas' through becoming administrator for the Special Trustees. At Guy's, the post of superintendent had long been one of its distinctive features. A member of the medical staff, the superintendent oversaw the administration of the hospital and the relationship with the medical school which was an unusual arrangement. During the 1960s as hospital administration became ever more complex, many of the post's executive responsibilities had passed to the clerk to the governors. But medical staff at Guy's were determined to hold on to the position in the new reorganisation and the post was included in the new structures under the name of clinical superintendent and had a place on the District Management Team.[3] St Thomas' had worked with PA Management Consultants to prepare its administrative structures for the new landscape and the Principal Management Team comprising the Clerk of the Governors, the Chairman of the Medical and Surgical Officers Committee, the Chief Nursing Officer, the Finance Officer and the Dean of the Medical School evolved into the District Management Team with the inclusion of the District Community Physician and some GPs, thereby representing the interests of the new district.[4] Despite the best efforts of the leadership in both institutions to retain continuities, some staff experienced the changes as catastrophic in subsuming institutional identity: 'in 1974, when the hospital was effectively destroyed by Godber's[5] actions...there was a strong move to remove the name "Guy's" completely from the hospital and to supplant it with simply "District General Hospital" and a number!' reflected one consultant.[6]

Patricia Moberly, who later served as chairman of the Guy's and St Thomas' NHS Foundation Trust, lived in the late 1960s with her husband and four children in Kennington and worked as a teacher. In 1971 she had joined Lambeth Council and challenged the proposed changes around hospital governance.

> What I do remember, is going and having an argument with David Owen (Under Secretary of State for Health and Social Security) and Barbara Castle (Secretary of State for Health and Social Security) about the abolition of governors... many of us thought that that was a pretty undemocratic, impersonal way of running hospitals... and telling David Owen that although the Keith Joseph plan had started to be discussed, it hadn't actually taken shape and appointments to positions had not been made, at the time of the February 1974 general election, and that he had plenty of time to stop it, and rethink it...He said, Oh, no, no, it's all being

implemented. I said, No, it isn't. We're actually down there on the ground and it's not being implemented. But…they went ahead and allowed it to happen, and they tagged on community health councils, as a kind of sop to local people, I think, because hospitals were losing their own governors and they wanted to have something a bit more focused on local communities.[7]

The new arrangements, for the first time, exposed hospital consultants to the vagaries of political control of healthcare. Barry Jackson who described his experience of applying to St Thomas' for a junior cardiac appointment in Chapter 2 became a consultant in 1973. He viewed St Thomas' as an 'invincible institution that had an absolutely long-term future' and was an institution considered by many staff to be '*the* hospital of the UK'. He reflected that at this point in time he had no sense that St Thomas' future was contingent on government health policy. Soon after the 1974 reorganisation, Walter Holland, then running the research unit, attended the Medical Staff Committee to explain its implications to consultant staff. 'Quite frankly, it didn't mean anything. We had just moved regions and so there were implications for rotations of junior medical staff…but it didn't really impinge on NHS staff in any great way,' reflected Barry. Five years later Barry was elected Chairman of the Medical Staff Committee and became involved in the management of the hospital. He realised that 'there were very significant changes ahead' and reflected that the consultant body had been 'incredibly sanguine' with little appreciation of the challenges of hospital management and the complex relationship with local and national authorities.[8]

That 1974 brought irrevocable change to Guy's and St Thomas' is illustrated by both institutions commissioning a written record of their post-war histories. The costs of this work were covered by the endowment funds at each institution. Robert Sharpington was invited to write a history of the management and administration of St Thomas' Hospital covering the period from 1927 to 1977. Rather than a nostalgic account of a golden past, the intention was for the history to be instrumental in the face of further change. In the Foreword, Sir John Prideaux, Chairman of the Special Trustees, stated his hope that the implications of the history would be 'taken to heart by those who create the new District Health Authorities and by those who become Members of them'. In his view, the 1974 structures revealed the need for management at local level that could contribute the same 'coherent purpose and sustained, disinterested leadership', as was exemplified in boards of governors.[9] At Guy's Hospital, David Stafford-Clark, a retired psychiatrist who had trained at Guy's, and worked as Director of the York Clinic between 1955 and 1971, was appointed to write a history.[10] This work was never finished because of a disagreement between Stafford-Clark and the Trustees about the critical nature of Stafford-Clark's interpretation of Guy's history.

Special Trustees

Planning for future developments was part of the DNA in both institutions. During the long lead-in time to the 1974 reorganisation, the institutions had taken the opportunity to anticipate and plan for the forthcoming changes.[11] One of the most important questions to be addressed was what should happen to teaching hospital endowment funds which had been given charitable status when the NHS was established in 1948. Apart from St Bartholomew's Hospital, Guy's and St Thomas' endowments were the largest in the UK with St Thomas' being the richer endowment. Guy's and St Thomas' had benefited considerably from these independent revenue streams which had underpinned developments in research, teaching, and care across the medical schools and the hospitals during the first decades of the NHS. Harry Burfoot, Clerk to the Governors at Guy's was Chairman of the Teaching Hospitals' Association and established a small working group to review the future of endowment funds. To keep control of the funds 'away from the Government', the group developed the concept of Special Trustees who would oversee the allocation and use of the funds. Harry formulated a proposal which was accepted 'reluctantly' by the Department of Health and Social Security with additional safeguards around the dismissal of trustees. The arrangements came into place in 1973 and gave the Secretary of State for Health the power to appoint Special Trustees to manage charitable property on behalf of hospital boards.[12] The core argument made by Harry and his group for the retention of endowment funds by hospitals was based on the significant public support for hospitals and an understanding of the motivations that lay behind public contributions.

> People over the years had given money to the teaching hospitals, for the benefit of those teaching hospitals not for anybody else's benefit…people who give money usually give because (a) they have a conscience, they have a hell of a lot of money and they want to start giving it away, and (b) they want their name to be remembered, and (c) they want to get some kudos from it. They want to give to something which is pretty important…Guy's name is a national name…Lambeth, Southwark, and Lewisham Area Health Authority means nothing to anybody – a chap who has given a £1 million can't talk to his buddies and say, I gave this money to the LSL AHA, as they would say what was that? Give it to Guy's and they know all about it.[13]

Managing endowment funds in the context of a national health system funded through taxation was a sensitive issue. When later questioned about the capital investment of the Guy's funds, Harry commented: 'we never value our investments for obvious purposes. If it looks too big, it riles people…The Fund at the moment [early 1980s] has a capital value of about £9 million – although that is a historic cost, in other words if you bought property in 1948 which cost £50,000, that property is still valued now at £50,000, although it may be worth half a million'.[14] There were initial uncertainties as to the appropriate remit of the endowment funds and at St Thomas', John Wyn Owen wrote a memorandum on the 'indivisibility' of the core functions of the institution across care, teaching, and research, and argued that it was as appropriate to support medical education as community services: 'the critical criterion was that the Trustees would not support the basic operation of the hospital or the medical school'.[15] Peter Lumsden had become involved with St Thomas' in the 1960s, first joining the Council of the Medical School and then becoming a governor. He had an illustrious career in finance, serving as Finance Director to the Morgan Crucible Group and the Inchcape Group. He became one of the Special Trustees and explained the fine distinctions surrounding the use of funds and the importance of supporting research even when outcomes were uncertain.

> They're there for the hospital, they're not there to subsidise the health service. Now, obviously there's times when those are rather blurred lines. You've also got to remember, when you're supporting research, you're really trying to decide what you think is a good idea to support, because you never know what the outcome's going to be…having looked into the eye of the person proposing it and you think they're competent and able, then you have to give them money to carry on with what they're doing to see what happens. Because we never know in research what's going to come out of it until the research has been completed, and it may take [several] years, depending on the type of the thing.[16]

Endowment funds enabled development at a scale that would have been unachievable elsewhere. At the end of the 1970s, for example, St Thomas' acquired Dr D Dumonde and his team from the Kennedy Institute to establish immunology as a major department: 'like you buy football players,' reflected John Wyn Owen.[17] Endowment funds also enabled improvements in the environment that were to the benefit of patients and staff. In 1972 at St Thomas', a History and Works of Art Committee was established with support from the endowment funds and began a programme of work to restore the hospital's collection of statues, paintings, and other objects including the Doulton Tile Pictures which were originally on the walls of the children's wards.[18] Patricia Mowbray had trained in art history and joined St Thomas' initially on a part-time basis to catalogue the art collections but became a full-time Art Historian in 1975, supported by the Special Trustees.

> I used to go into a ward with a barrow load of works and say, Sister, would you care to have some art? And they would say, Oh we don't want any of that modern stuff. And I would say, I see, and I'd find some very simple painting of a cow in a field and then they'd say, Oh that's nice. Then I'd go a little further and I'd get down to, Well you see if the person is sitting over here in a wheelchair, they can't see anything in that picture as it doesn't show up, but if you get [a picture with] striking colour, warmth and ships say, you can see it from a distance. So I'd show them the difference between the cow in the field there and then a very striking new kind of vibrant [picture] and they'd begin to come round and eventually I would find I got every picture I wanted to get up in that ward.[19]

Tooting Bec Hospital, which provided mental health services, had joined St Thomas' Health District in 1974 and underwent an extensive programme of upgrading its buildings and grounds. Patricia was given a 'generous budget' to buy and install works of art in the wards and dayrooms, although safety concerns after a 'much-loved nurse' had been stabbed to death by an inmate meant that she was protected by a guard whilst she worked. The initiative at Tooting Bec led to patients receiving in-patient care for mental health at St

Thomas' Hospital being invited to select a picture to be hung on the wall opposite their bed. When Patricia asked the consultant for advice in communicating with these patients, the reply was, 'simply treat the patient as you would any normal person'.[20]

During the same period the Guy's Joint Consultative Staffs Committee was asked to create a Staff Club that would serve as a meeting place for staff to exchange views on 'workloads, the price of tea, conditions at different hospitals, attitudes and ideas'.[21] It spoke to the increasing size and complexity of the institution and the need to build closer bonds between staff. Given the pressure on space across buildings, an area was eventually identified in the basement of the old Superintendent's House, situated under the West Wing of Guy's House, which dated from 1780. Plans were drawn up which involved providing electricity, ventilation, heating, air conditioning and cooling, and plumbing work amounting to around £25k. These were cut back to around £20k and the proposal was taken to the Endowments Committee who agreed to fund the scheme. The location of the work and the sharp rises in building costs meant that only one firm was willing to tender for the work and submitted an estimate of £28k. To cover the additional costs, the Committee secured an interest-free loan of £7.5k from the brewers, Whitbread's, with the agreement that they would provide drinks for the bar. Staff fundraising activities were planned to raise the additional £500 and the Endowments Committee agreed to underwrite the loan from Whitbread's.[22] Many hospitals across the NHS would have faced similar challenges as the size of workforces grew, but without the benefit of endowment funds had no means to redress them.

Importantly, keeping control of the endowment funds enabled the institutions to retain some of the confidence that derived from their autonomy in the pre-1974 era. Sir Patrick Nairne, Permanent Secretary to the Department of Health, visited St Thomas' for a dinner in 1976/77 and Sir John Prideaux, Chairman of the Special

Trustees wasted little time in reminding him that as a teaching hospital, St Thomas' had a tradition of 'not going with the grain,' adding: 'we will go with the grain when it appears to us that it is the right thing to do. But don't forget that we've been here a long time and therefore with our endowment we will decide'.[23] Between 1974 and 1984, endowment funds contributed to around £25 million of investments and enabled the institution to move in new directions with a freedom that most other institutions, particularly those outside London, could only dream of. St Thomas' alumni moving to work in other parts of the health service reflected that it was very difficult to secure organisational and clinical research and innovation with a 'pittance of endowments'.[24]

Developing service management and clinical research

The future direction of health services management was anticipated in 1972 at St Thomas' with the appointment of John Wyn Owen as assistant clerk with a brief to inform planning processes with research evidence. John, born in Bangor, North Wales, had read Geography at the University of Cambridge and began training in NHS administration at the King's Fund in 1964. Whilst later working at the University Hospital Group in Cardiff, John was invited by the King's Fund to arrange a programme on health services for a visiting group of 25 Americans at short notice. He later found that he had been chosen because he was viewed as their best trainee to date. 'I [rang] top people saying, this is not a matter for negotiation. I need you to speak at this prestigious conference between the hours of X and Y and this is the topic.' It led to an invitation to spend six months touring the US with 25 institutional hosts and John used his time to research comparative US and UK approaches to running healthcare as a business. On return to the UK, he was invited to join St Thomas' as assistant clerk working on the commissioning and implementation of health service research.[25] Despite the wrench of moving from his beloved Wales to London, the offer was 'too much to resist'. John found St Thomas' to be a unique place with eminent medical staff who enjoyed thriving practices on Harley Street, and numerous Royal Appointments. The Queen was Patron, and the Chairman of the Board of Governors was the Chairman of the National Westminster Bank: 'you were dealing with the premier division of people right across the spectrum'. John found it to be a collegiate institution with a shared focus on achievement and a strong historical identity perpetuated through the memory of figures such as Florence Nightingale. The sense of having the best people permeated all aspects of the institutional life, including an exchange programme for chefs with the Ritz Hotel which resulted in the hospital catering team winning international awards. Marcel Jacquemin who worked at St Thomas' for 37 years in the kitchens remembered winning 'silver cups and medals' and when Marcel's father became Head Chef, he won the International Chef of the Year Award and 'was plastered all over the world'.[26] John's view was that 'wherever you looked, you had excellence, or outstanding performance'.[27]

The 1974 reorganisation required the administration 'to think, plan, and operate in a wider context than hitherto, so as to encompass both community aspects of health care, as well as purely hospital-based services, functions, and activities' and this put greater demands on the managerial capability of staff.[28] John described the changes in his role as 'a shift of responsibility from institutional management to having responsibilities for the health of a defined community of 200,000 people in West Lambeth'.[29] St Thomas' commissioned PA Management Consultants to support the introduction of an in-house management training programme which launched in June 1975 and integrated the most up to date management theory and practice. The outcomes were noted in an editorial in the *International Management Journal*: 'in an era of steeply rising medical care costs a London hospital group has actually managed to reduce expenditure by adopting some basic principles of business management'. Accounting and cost management systems had been integrated into administration since the 1960s but there had been little impact on day-to-day medicine and nursing. One of the aims of the new training was to raise fiscal awareness across the staff. 'As a nurse, we have never had to think about money. If we wanted anything we asked for it and usually got it,' noted Ward Sister Gillian Hurst. Yet increasing financial pressures made it imperative that everyone involved in healthcare needed to understand 'what it means to have a budget,' said John Wyn Owen. Nevertheless, some aspects of care could not be measured and rationalised: 'I can tell you how long it takes to give an injection but I cannot measure how much emotional time I may need to spend with somebody…You can guess what might happen if there will be a death. But people do not die to order,' commented Ward Sister Gillian Hurst.[30]

Clinical research became increasingly prominent during this period and Guy's showcased this shift: '[through] appointing academic heads of specialities in the hospital, in a small way at first, for example gastroenterology and nephrology, and that process continued. So, if you like, the academic aspect of life permeated into hospital and clinical activity much more evidently than it would in the older type of division between the academic departments … and the proper doctors outside those walls who really did the proper medicine and surgery,' remembered Gwyn Williams who joined Guy's in the early 1970s as a renal consultant.[31] Guy's alumnus, Professor Stewart Cameron, had set up the renal unit in the 1960s, and in 1971 Cyril Chantler, also Guy's alumnus, was appointed as consultant paediatrician and tasked with developing services for renal failure in children. Cyril's experience illustrates the challenges of establishing research as integral to clinical practice. The Evelina Hospital for Sick Children, founded in 1869 by Baron Ferdinand de Rothschild after his wife, Evelina, and their baby had died in premature labour, had joined the Guy's group of hospitals when the NHS was established in 1948. The Evelina had a 'special atmosphere' and was 'known and trusted' by the local community.[32] James Houston, Dean of the Medical and Dental School, had assured Cyril at the interview that laboratory facilities, staff, and funding would be made available to support his research on low growth in children with renal failure: 'we were keeping these children alive on kidney machines and transplanting them in the expectation that they would stay alive... but we had this huge problem of growth failure which was terribly damaging to them and their families,' remembered Cyril. When he returned from working for the Medical Research Council in America to take up the post, he found 'empty space, no equipment, and no salary for technicians, or scientists'. He queried the situation with the Dean who acknowledged giving the assurance but stated there was 'nothing he could do about it' – Cyril would have to go and fundraise himself. The Dean then asked Cyril whether he had considered moving to Great Ormond Street Children's Hospital because it was a postgraduate institution and funded to do research through the University of London: 'Guy's is here to teach clinical medicine to the students, we are not here to do research, the pre-clinical doctors do some research to keep themselves happy but that's not what we do,' added the Dean.[33] That held true for earlier decades when the Medical and Dental School's income from external research grants stood at £2,250, but by the early 1970s it had risen significantly to £34k. Cyril was part of a new generation who were committed to creating a science-base for teaching and practice. He was a founder member of the British Association for Paediatric Nephrology and Guy's became one of the first dedicated paediatric haemodialysis units in the UK.[34]

During the mid-1970s the original Evelina Hospital was closed and reinstated in Guy's Tower, and Cyril and colleagues again had to wage battles to preserve the unique 'ethos' and identity of the Evelina: 'I always used to call it The Evelina and we used to get phone calls from the Department of Health saying, we don't have this hospital called

The Evelina on our books any longer, I used to say, no, it's called the Evelina Children's Unit, but it's a children's hospital,' said Cyril. One of the critical issues at the planning stage concerned the children's casualty department. The paediatricians were determined that there should be a children's casualty department with its own separate entrance and waiting area. This was to save children and families from the 'horrendous' experience of attending an adult Accident and Emergency department. The agreement was made but as the building evolved Cyril 'got wind' that there had been a change of plan: 'I knew once we'd moved into Guy's, if we didn't have it, we'd never get it.' The following week the *South London Gazette* bore a headline stating: 'doctors refuse to leave Evelina Hospital'. Cyril was summoned to see Dr Philip Halliwell, the Medical Superintendent: 'He said, Cyril, are you responsible for this? I said, yes, Dr Halliwell, I am. He said, well, it's disgraceful because it's not true! Oh, I said, in that case I'm very sorry but I was told that you'd said that we couldn't have the area. He said, well you can have the area. I said, fine, will you phone the *South London Gazette,* or will I?'[35]

Working cultures

The 1970s was a time of immense social and political change which included new attempts to address longstanding inequities through legislation including the 1970 Equal Pay Act which came into force in 1975, the 1975 Sex Discrimination Act, and the 1976 Race Relations Act. These broader changes played out across the institutions, reshaping working practices and staff relationships.

Natalie Tiddy trained in nursing at St Thomas' and had joined the nursing administration during the implementation of the 1967 Salmon Report on nurse staffing structures. She describes how she worked to develop consistency across all nursing appointments within the St Thomas' Health District and set up a personnel department.

There were now chief nurses, senior nursing officers, nursing officers...I was made a nursing officer in the department of nursing. The nursing officer at the Royal Waterloo Hospital had become ill so I was asked if I'd go and manage the Waterloo Hospital [which joined St Thomas' Hospital Group in 1948] ...anyway, I managed that for six months while this person was ill. I then came back. It then struck me, being in the administration department, that there was no common area for the recruitment of nursing staff at all these hospitals. We were called St Thomas' Health District, but every hospital functioned separately, and there was a need to draw together the whole appointment structure. So, I spoke to the then Chief Nurse, Sheila Garratt, and I laid out my ideas, wrote out what I thought needed to be done, and she said, fine, you sort it out. So as a nursing officer I developed the department of nursing personnel, and over time we centralised the whole recruitment and appointment process of all those hospitals. So, it was the Royal Waterloo, South Western, Tooting Bec Hospital, St Thomas', and the Grosvenor. That took quite a lot of negotiation because there were people in post who felt that they were doing the job particularly well and why did I think anybody could do it better than them. But it necessitated drawing up common procedures as much as anything else so that the same application form for St Thomas' Health District was used on each site, the same sorts of contracts were written...I never had a contract when I was a nursing officer, or indeed, when I was a staff nurse. Yes, you got a letter, which is the same as a contract, but it never talked about money or conditions of service or hours of work. You just knew what they were. So, I set up the nursing personnel by myself and a secretary, and it grew.[36]

Amidst the changes, longstanding institutions such as the consultants' dining room with 'white-coated waiters serving the food' retained its importance as a hub for networking around patient care. Richard Thompson was appointed consultant gastroenterologist at St Thomas' in 1972, setting up a new research laboratory and developing clinical practice. He reflected on the benefits of the dining room.

> It was extremely positive for care in the sense you could relate about patients, talk to other consultants, and it was very good for morale…It was [consultants'] place of contact with the hospital. Because in those days, of course, the consultants didn't – unless they were academic – have offices in the hospital. They had a secretary that they would go and dictate letters to, and they had the consultant dining room for tea or lunch.[37]

Eddyna Danso came to the UK from Sierra Leone, West Africa in 1967 to join her parents who had migrated a few years previously. After finishing grammar school, she spotted an advert in the *Sun* newspaper to train at Guy's as a theatre technician. She was successful at interview and began in September 1973.

> You were paid while you were training, which was important to me, because my parents could not afford to send me to university, or to support me to study…Guy's, it was very white, even then it was still white Britain…living in the East End, you were used to seeing Black and Asian people around. But when I came to Guy's it was very white, very male-orientated…coming in as a trainee theatre technician, again, that area was very male-orientated…a lot of the theatre technicians were men…sometimes felt I was treated differently, but I enjoyed my training because, one thing that sort of spurred me on, not to get despondent, to know

> I could do it, was because the head of the training school
> was a Black Jamaican man [George Wedderburn]… But I
> must say, most of the consultants, and the anaesthetists,
> and the surgeons were gentlemen. They would rather not
> acknowledge you…You were just ignored.

Eddyna qualified in 1975 and chose to work on the surgical rather
than the anaesthetic side and became one of the first operating
department assistants in the hospital.[38] She remembers colleagues
making racist jokes when TV series such as *Love Thy Neighbour* –
which has since been criticised for portraying racial tensions in a
way which normalised both anti-black and anti-white prejudices –
were playing in the coffee room: 'I never laughed it off. If I didn't
find it funny…I would say to individuals, I don't find that funny…I
only challenged one individual, and I still remember it…someone
was there who stopped me, because this individual went on with his
abuse, and if I hadn't been stopped, it would have got physical.'

Eddyna spent time at Evelina Hospital during her training and
described how a combination of racism and nursing hierarchical
cultures led to her being ignored by the sister in charge as she was
instructed to communicate only with the staff nurse. At the end of
the week 'I went up to her, even though she hadn't spoken to me all
week. Sister, I said, Sister, I'll be late back from lunch because I need
to go to Guy's to collect my wages. And she was stunned. Are you
speaking to me? she said. Go and speak to my staff nurse'. The tables
were turned a few years later when the Evelina was relocated to
Guy's Tower. By this point Eddyna was 'qualified, well-established,
well-known, and confident'. To begin with the Evelina nurses 'were
like fish out of water. They didn't know any of the staff' and Eddyna
came across the sister who had treated her with such disdain in
the changing room: 'I remember you, Sister, I'll never forget you',
said Eddyna. But within a few weeks the more integrated ways of

working in teams took effect and Eddyna and the sister became firm friends.[39]

By the late 1970s, staff were becoming more diverse. William Tatton Brown, former chief architect at the Department of Health and Social Security, who wrote a detailed account of his stay as an in-patient at St Thomas', mentioned a Portuguese cleaner, and a Thai nurse who worked on the ward he stayed in.[40]

Royal openings

Guy's and St Thomas' had established comprehensive post-war rebuilding programmes and 1976 marked milestones on both sites. At Guy's, the completion of the Tower coincided with the 250th anniversary of the admission of the first patient to the hospital and a two-day celebration took place in May. The Tower was opened by Her Majesty, Queen Elizabeth II and other events included a Thanksgiving Service at Southwark Cathedral; the Annual Meeting of the Nurses' League; a scientific meeting; and many social events including a formal dinner and sports events. Guy's Hospital Gazette published a commemorative volume, *Guy's Hospital: 250 Years*. Underlying the pride and delight in the long history of achievements as 'a world famous institution' was apprehension and a sense that the community was standing 'on the brink of vast changes in our hospital life; certainly as important and as far reaching as the original foundation of Guy's as a deed of pity and charity': the dissolution of Boards of Governors was a stark symbol of the division between past, present, and an uncertain future.[41] Lord Russell Brock, alumnus of Guy's and pioneer of open-heart surgery, gave the oration which referenced the original split from St Thomas': 'Quarrelling now arose between the staffs of the two hospitals. Much of the trouble seems to have arisen from a certain feeling of jealousy on the part of St Thomas' staff that this upstart hospital of Thomas Guy had reached such eminence and at the expense of St Thomas.'[42] He concluded with the hope that the identity of the hospital would be preserved and 'will not, as a result of reorganisation, be called merely the District Hospital of Southwark but will retain its true name that recalls throughout this country and the whole world the memory of the great contributions that have come from it in its 250 years of existence and of service'.[43] Some comfort may have been taken from the Queen's affirmation that: 'I am sure that Guy's will go on making the best possible use of its buildings and medical knowledge, within the framework of the National Health Service, and, above all, will retain the caring approach to its work for the community which has been the one constant characteristic of its history'.[44]

In November 1976 the new North Wing at St Thomas' was opened by the Queen. The rebuilding not just upgraded facilities but enabled the hospital to better fulfil its new responsibilities to the community: 'As part of St Thomas' Health District, the new buildings will be a vital element not only in the making of a better hospital service for the people of West Lambeth but also in the provision for them of a total service embodying every aspect of their health care throughout their lives. In the development of this provision the traditions of service to the local communities of Lambeth Hospital are going to be combined with those of St Thomas' Hospital to its further enrichment...the new buildings will sustain and even strengthen St Thomas' place as a national hospital.'[45] The event encouraged staff embroiled in the challenges of the moment to draw sustenance from embracing the longer history of the institution. G Wetherly-Mein, Professor of Haematology, summed up the value of the Royal visit.

> The morale of the National Health Service is low and the teaching hospitals, in particular, are being criticised for being too big, too expensive, too sophisticated, too old-fashioned and, perhaps, even too good. In addition, the bureaucratic paperchase, a lunacy of Homeric stature, increasingly distracts and dismays all those responsible

for the actual care of patients. Even this Foundation of St Thomas', experienced in survival since about 1215, was beginning to feel uncertain of its purpose and its value. In some extraordinary way the Queen's visit made the important things seem important and the tiresome things trivial. We felt better and are grateful for it.[46]

Growing financial pressures

The Royal openings were light moments in a difficult period as the oil crisis, the International Monetary Fund bailout, and industrial action across the public sector intensified pressure on health services and the balancing of budgets. More broadly, the growing costs of the NHS in the context of an ageing population and huge expansion in medical technologies were creating 'dilemmas of choice' that forced Guy's and St Thomas' to engage more deeply with the application of economic principles to health service management.[47] Both institutions had taken note of the King's Fund 1973 report on *Accounting for Health*.[48] Guy's and St Thomas' were particularly affected by the attempts to distribute funding more equitably across the NHS. For the first decades in the NHS, the institutions had received funding allocations according to their historical patterns of spending and as Chapter 2 showed, these had been supplemented from the endowment funds and successful bids for capital funding. But there was growing political concern that this mechanism of funding distribution created unevenness which translated into unequal provision for patients.[49] The 1974 reorganisation proved decisive as it enabled comparison of expenditure on populations in different authorities as for the first time, hospital and community health expenditure was brought together under the new AHAs. Hospitals were required to submit detailed statistics on activities and the pressure to justify beds and budgets is suggested by a handwritten note on the cover of a 1973 report by the South East Metropolitan Regional Hospital Board Management Services Division which compiled hospital statistics:

'Guy's Hospital very fishy. 100% of occupancy for all beds except paediatrics.' These comparisons revealed how the disparities between areas in the same region were even greater than those across regions. Malcolm Forsythe had trained in medicine at Guy's. He was Area Medical Officer for Kent AHA between 1974 and 1978 and then joined the South East Metropolitan Regional Hospital Board, in 1978, as Regional Medical Officer. The region had had no significant new buildings since 1948 and was struggling to address the problems resulting from the demographic shift of people from London to the Home Counties which required services to be reconfigured to meet needs in new places. Malcolm was under no doubt that change was needed:

> Within our region we had over-provided London districts
> and we had under-provided counties, Kent and Sussex, and
> to go with that we had appalling primary care in London,
> we had our own mental health scandal and then we wanted
> to rationalise the regional specialities.[50]

Malcolm joined the Resource Allocation Working Party (RAWP) set up by the Department of Health in 1975 and other members included Walter Holland, Director of the Social Medicine and Health Services Research Unit at St Thomas'. Encouraged by Brian Abel Smith, Chair of the Unit's Advisory Committee, Walter had done some initial work around resource distribution, taking an epidemiological approach to the health needs of Lambeth which led to David Owen, Minister of State for Health, inviting him to join RAWP.[51] The RAWP group developed a new formula for allocating NHS funding according to need and published its report, *Sharing Resources for Health in England*, in September 1976. South East Thames Region was advised that as a result of RAWP, it would lose between £11 million to £13 million from its £100 million annual budget. This translated into a £3 million loss for each hospital and the news made front page headlines in the *Daily Telegraph* on Friday 26 November.

David Loshak, health correspondent, noted that the proposals for Lambeth, Southwark, and Lewisham area seemed the 'most drastic' of all and since staff salaries accounted for around 80 per cent of the AHA budget, enforced job losses seemed inevitable.[52]

Ron Kerr, later to become Chief Executive of Guy's and St Thomas' NHS Foundation Trust, began his career in health services management by working in capital planning at the Manchester Regional Hospital Board. He moved to London in 1977 as services planner in the North East Thames region and reflected on the challenges of reconfiguring health services in London in a context of industrial unrest and clashes around financial restrictions.

> London...needed to consolidate its hospital settings. Certainly, needed to modernise its estate. Probably needed to think about better integrating primary care and secondary care...I have this memory of us gradually beginning to absorb into the major centres the plethora of small units which existed across all elements of London... there was a lot of building around London to consolidate and improve the estate of what was pretty run down in many ways. So, I think that was the general picture. As initially a planner and then somebody running hospitals there was the beginnings of a real focus on efficiency and the beginnings of proper comparison between performance of different organisations in some more material way than existed before...The other two things which of course were material in that period was, one, the industrial relations environment that we operated, which was really pretty severe in the late '70s and early '80s with all the noise around public sector reflecting the divisions in society at the time, and a significant part of the responsibilities of anybody running a hospital at that time was dealing with those issues of HR, industrial relations in a strike-hit

environment or one where there was a lot of debate. [And two] health authority meetings being held in really quite confrontational, quite hostile environments...Lambeth, Southwark, and Lewisham having quite a reputation from that point of view as a health authority which was quite robust in its support for perhaps what might have been seen as a more left of centre view of the world than some other places.[53]

Balancing budgets was a major source of contention. Guy's and St Thomas' had demonstrated adaptability in developing rationalisation plans that aimed to develop services whilst saving costs but by the late 1970s tensions were running high. St Thomas' finance department was understood to be highly skilled in 'providing accounts which seemed to reflect St Thomas' in a very favourable light...there was a certain amount of obfuscation of some of the data that was supplied to the region about what was going on at St Thomas' on staffing matters and finance matters and so on'.[54] Guy's too were adjusting to financial stringency. The Medical Committee was used to seeking funding for new developments and since 1948 the institution had enjoyed access, first to the Ministry of Health and then the Department of Health and Social Security to lobby for discretionary funding. Cyril Chantler remembered a meeting in the late 1970s when the finance director attended and said, 'I'm afraid we have no money this meeting for developments and we all said, what? ...then the gap widened between what we wanted to do, because science was providing more and more possibilities, and the funding which had stopped.'[55]

Rising inflation had caused the Labour Government to impose pay restraints on the public sector beginning in 1975. In 1976 the Callaghan Government had obtained a loan from the International Monetary Fund to help address the rising inflation but trade union resistance to this action led to widespread public sector strikes. By 1978 NHS staff had experienced a 19 per cent drop in real wages and from October 1978 a national wave of strikes across many sectors created what became known as 'the Winter of Discontent', accompanied by deep snow and blizzards. Across London AHAs were faced with the choice of maintaining services across districts or preserving national and regional specialties that fell within the AHA and the pressures encouraged militant responses.

Through the 1970s Lambeth Council had been 'a fairly middle of the road, rather proud Council with some very good senior officers, forward thinking in many ways but very well respected,' said Patricia Moberly. The pressures of 1979, however, led to 'a sort of militant takeover' and she was not re-elected: 'In fact, I was dumped. Probably the best thing that ever happened to me, because I would have hated it, as it turned out.' But she expressed frustration with people who conflated her period as councillor with the later militant era: 'I always have a go when people talk about the terrible, radical left Labour people. I think, actually you're thinking of people after us, not of us at all. We were perfectly normal. But Lambeth acquired that reputation, but not at the period when I was a councillor.'[56] Barry Jackson also recollected strong left-wing views on the Council which were 'anti-Thomas' and spoke 'very strongly against the place and considered it elitist'.[57]

In the early summer of 1979 John Wyn Owen, then District Administrator for St Thomas' Health District who also sat on the Lambeth, Southwark, and Lewisham AHA, brought a senior group of St Thomas' clinicians and administrators together to discuss future strategies. The workshop was held at Leeds Castle, a Grade 1 listed building with origins dating from 1119, a few miles outside Maidstone. The aim of the event was to 'establish a broad, shared vision of what the District is striving towards' by asking questions such as: what has St Thomas' accomplished that is distinctive and special to itself? what are the essential strengths that it has to preserve and renew? what qualities will St Thomas' wish to be renowned in the future? to what threats is St Thomas' most vulnerable? what are the barriers and opportunities? The focus was to develop 'thoughtful opinions and philosophies', not an action plan.[58] Healthcare planning teams were asked to set out the issues across acute specialities, community healthcare, maternity services, services for children, and mental health. Representatives from the Community Health Council and the Director of Social Services for the London Borough of Lambeth also joined some sessions. Brian Abel-Smith, Professor of Economics at the London School of Economics, acted as assessor for the event. Brian had a long association with St Thomas', serving as governor between 1957 and 1968. His closing address noted St Thomas' strengths: an increased rate of manpower compared to national averages; savings from hospital closures; and benefits from the Revenue Consequences of Capital Schemes.[59] The challenges arising in the future, noted Brian, were likely to come from the continuing population decline in the inner-city areas, the inflexibility of hospital plant, and increasing competition for patients in London. Outcomes were decided around the institution's immediate and longer term priorities: agreement to open talks with Guy's about the merger of the medical schools; acceptance of the move to the South East Thames region; adoption of a deprived district; a continued focus on the elderly, the mentally ill, and the consolidation of services; and the need to address social cohesion in local communities, in light of racial tensions, especially around Brixton, high levels of unemployment, and the lack of educational opportunities for local young people who were not qualified enough to join St Thomas' workforce.

But within weeks of the workshop in August 1979 the immediate issues of cash limits across the Lambeth, Southwark, and Lewisham AHA came to a head. The Conservatives had won the May 1979 General Election with a manifesto that promised to reduce public spending and Patrick Jenkin was appointed Secretary of State for Social Services. When Lambeth, Southwark, and Lewisham AHA was presented with evidence about the impact on patients of cutting back speciality services, they refused to implement cuts to ensure the budget remained within the set cash limits.[60] Jenkin was notified of the AHA's decision that 'it did not intend to remain within its cash limits' and he intervened rapidly and appointed Sir John Prideaux, Chair of St Thomas' Special Trustees, and Miss Nuttall as Commissioners to take over the responsibilities of the AHA. The Commissioners were given the same functions and powers as the AHA and maintained the relationship with the South East Thames Regional Health Authority.[61] Barry Jackson, surgeon at St Thomas', had been appointed chairman of the Medical Staff Committee and member of the District Management Team shortly before the crisis. He was called to meet with the commissioners and remembers 'being cross-questioned pretty closely…about what was going on. I realised then that things were going to have to change'.[62] The decision was challenged by the three London boroughs and in February 1980, a High Court judge ruled that the action was unlawful, causing the Tories enormous embarrassment. Powers were returned to the AHA which 'accepted that it was their responsibility to live within the cash limits set by the Government and the Regional Health Authority'.[63] The 1980 Health Services Act which created District Health Authorities introduced a legal requirement for health authorities and health boards to manage expenditure within the set cash limits. Savings were eventually achieved locally through bed closures and rationalisation programmes in support services.[64]

Patients and technologies

Through the 1970s new treatments including dialysis and transplantation first introduced in the 1960s became established as everyday treatments. Renal units had been set up at both Guy's and St Thomas', and Liz Jenkins joined the renal unit at Guy's in 1969 after qualifying as a nurse at St Thomas'.

When I went to the renal unit at Guy's in 1969, I came across many nurses from elsewhere. Within my first week I received a patient for dialysis from one of the wards, to discover he was still lying on the stretcher canvas that he had been to theatre on the day before. I therefore found some screens, a bowl and soap, and rolled him off the canvas and was washing his back and rubbing his bum, when the sister in charge of the unit came to see what I was doing. Instead of the praise I expected, her comment was, 'stop doing that, you didn't come here to nurse, you came to learn to dialyse'. This made me realise that not everyone senior to me understood what nursing is about. I did learn to dialyse quite well, and I never stopped nursing.

Despite that tricky start, Liz relished working in the unit.

It was like going into a sort of time warp because here was a group of people who truly worked together properly. A place where nurses were respected for the job they did, were listened to, and had the autonomy and authority that I don't think many nurses have even now. This was partly to do with the fact that we were doing pioneering work, and the doctors, nurses, and technicians were learning together all the time. Also, we had little interaction with nursing administration who did not understand what we were doing and so kept well out of our way. That and the fear of hepatitis I have to say helped. So, we worked as a real team. There was a long period of time when we had the lowest sickness and absence rate of any hospital department. That was simply because if one of us didn't turn up for work there wasn't anyone else who could do the job, so although we employed agency nurses, they were long-term and became part of the team.[65]

Wyndham Lloyd-Davies, urologist at St Thomas', undertook the first peritoneal dialysis there in 1964 working with kidney specialist Norman Jones: 'there was, in fact, a mechanical dialyser sitting in the corridor gathering dust and we got hold of it and got it cleaned and sorted out and we started the haemodialysis programme here with that and it all went from very small beginnings'.[66] Dialysis was a revolutionary treatment saving patients death from kidney failure: 'we had seven people on regular dialysis going through that pretty well non-stop little unit, but what I do remember is that when we had our, and of course methods were nothing like as sophisticated then as they are now, but when we had our 21st birthday party as a renal unit, five of those seven were there, 21 years later. That, I think, is one of my happiest memories,' recalled Norman Jones.[67]

But resource limitations meant that clinicians had to make difficult decisions about which patients should be offered treatments.

> I was on a committee which decided who would be dialysed and there were very strict criteria of age, of social situation, families. I remember very well a lady who was a year or so older than our criteria, but we took her on, because she had a daughter, and many years later, she was transplanted and survived it. I met her in the corridor, oh, about I think ten years after she had been transplanted, and she came up and said, you won't remember me, Mr Lloyd-Davies, I said, Oh, Mrs Smith, your name is engraved on my heart! And she said, I'm a grandmother, and the reason that we had put her on the programme was her daughter who was 11. She had done very well on dialysis and been transplanted and now had got her first grandchild. This brought it home that this was a very important aspect of trying to make these very hard decisions.[68]

Marianne Vennegoor joined the St Thomas' renal unit shortly after it was created in 1968 as its dietician. In the beginning the renal unit was part of the intensive care unit but over the early period it moved to Lambeth Hospital, a short walk away from St Thomas', then in 1976 returned to the South Wing. Having a dietician on the renal team was innovative and enabled dietary advice and regimes (kidney patients were not able to tolerate normal or high levels of protein in their diets) to be fully integrated into treatment programmes. Indeed, said Marianne, 'if the patients were able to stick to a diet well enough before dialysis started, then that was an indicator of how well the patient would do on dialysis'.

> My little office was at the spiral staircase, and the sister in charge had her office there too, and it was also the nurses' staffroom…I don't know how many dialysis stations we had there. There must have been at least ten or 12, and we were working together with the nurses, with the dieticians, with the patients, with the technicians, with the social workers; so we had quite a good time as a group, because the patients were our friends too…we became very patient-orientated because you saw them every time they came on dialysis, more or less, so they became your friends; and that's why they are still my friends – the ones I've kept in contact with.

The patients hugely appreciated the close relationships they enjoyed with staff.

> They were quite naughty, because they had to dialyse during the weekdays, because you needed access to support at the hospital, and during the weekends the unit was closed. So, they would dialyse in the weekend all the same! You know, and not tell us.[69]

Marianne worked in the unit for more than 45 years and one of her long-standing patients was Brian Marchant. Brian worked in the Civil Service and in 1969 at the age of 32 he began to suffer from blurred vision. He initially attended Guy's but was transferred to St Thomas' because the Guy's dialysis unit was full. After various tests he was diagnosed with kidney failure and put on a special protein-restricted diet that had been developed in the 1960s because kidney patients could not tolerate normal or high levels of protein.

> You couldn't get everything readily from the shops…it was difficult at times to keep to the diet, because of the way you had to do your cooking…was more or less cooking for two different types of meals…and the wife would have something entirely different as well.

As well as the restricted diet, Brian had to limit his fluid consumption which was particularly hard in the summer months and after collapsing at work he began dialysis which was 30 hours a week and was split into three overnight ten-hour sessions.

> I managed to keep down a job, which meant dialysing overnight in Lambeth and then carrying on to work the next morning and then going home at the end of the day, so it worked out all right. Although I didn't see home much in those days.

Brian read to pass the time or watched TV, but the reception was often unreliable because of the interference from the dialysis machines. In 1970 he underwent his first transplant but there were persistent problems which led to him spending seven months in isolation on a side ward. Options for activities were limited and Brian remembered doing a lot of occupational therapy which involved 'making the usual mosaic ashtrays and that sort of thing'.[70] He eventually returned to dialysis and in 1972 he underwent a second transplant. This time it was successful, and he remained in good health with regular clinic check-ups until his death in 2016 aged 79. (The image on this book's cover shows Brian in the dialysis unit c.1970.)

Francis Tibbles was referred to Norman Jones as a teenager in the 1960s and remembers being 'patient number seven', in the dialysis programme.

> I was lucky because there were other guys there who didn't get to go on dialysis and must have died…I can only assume that was to do with age, perhaps parental support, and maybe physical fitness as well, that they thought perhaps I would be a good candidate to cope with it, because I was always playing sport so I was always fairly fit, until the year before when I didn't have the energy to do that…At some point during that time they decided that I was ideal for home dialysis…by that time I think they'd opened the new dialysis unit over in Lambeth Hospital, in a new purpose-built building at the far end. So, I used to go in there for training, and once they were happy, I went home, and you had support on the phone. If there was any problems with the Cambridge machines you could ring up somebody from the Cambridge company and they would drive, even in the middle of the night, and sort out the problem if they could. If they couldn't then obviously the back-up position was in the car and over to St Thomas'.

Francis thrived on the programme and was able to resume sports, playing table tennis and cricket. The only aspect he had to be careful of was to protect the shunt in his arm which was the access point for dialysis. He worked in the Civil Service and did his dialysis overnight for ten hours, three nights a week which was reduced to seven hours with the benefit of new machines from 1977 onwards. Sleeping patterns, however, could be disturbed because at times problems with the exchange rate of the various chemicals caused low blood pressure: 'you'd have to change various dials on the machine to increase the fluid back into you'. Maintaining the dialysis machines and equipment also required a lot of time.

> It was hard work, particularly for my mother, because my mother had to help me build those machines, strip them down, help wash and clean them. That prevented her from really having a full-time job…You had to put all your dialysis equipment, lines, needles, syringes, everything, all the stuff you had to go in your water softener. You'd lost half your bedroom to dialysis equipment, and even your wardrobe had gone. So, everything had to be in its place, because if it wasn't it would take you twice as long to get ready, and in an emergency if you wanted something quickly you knew where it was.

In 1978 Francis decided that he would put himself forward for transplantation because dialysis made it very difficult to develop relationships.

> It's very difficult having relationships with the opposite sex, and you tend to steer clear…Luckily for me my sister was actually a perfect match. We look very similar. Same height, same sort of build, same colour hair. It was the perfect match, so we went ahead. She had all the interviews to make sure she was okay with this…it all went really well, and we haven't really looked back. I had no real problems since the transplant…I was able to go and do all the sports I ever wanted to do.

Francis met his wife in 1986 and they went on to have a son 'so all in all it's been a very good family life'.[71]

Conclusion

For Guy's and St Thomas', the 1970s was a tough and turbulent decade. The loss of Boards of Governors was felt keenly by the institutions and the new era was sharply defined by the difficulties of managing service development and medical innovations in the context of reduced budgets. As the decade ended, the merger of the medical schools was on the horizon, as was a growing realisation that the unprecedented financial pressures would require a new approach. Nevertheless, the institutions' long history of surviving earlier challenges, especially around the financing and development of the hospitals, had created an institutional capacity to look to anticipate change, and wherever possible, to use it as an opportunity for institutional advancement. Further afield, the 'widespread concern' about the NHS had led to the setting up of a Royal Commission on the National Health Service, chaired by Sir Alec Merrison in the wake of the 1974 Reorganisation. In submitted evidence, Walter Holland, Robert Maxwell, and John Wyn Owen described themselves as: 'three individuals connected with St Thomas' Health District and Medical School, who are committed to a concept of the National Health Service, troubled by its current problems, and concerned to improve it. Our views are influenced by the fact that we all have international interests and experience'. Their three key messages were to: remove the Area tier not solely on the basis of cost but 'because of the frustration and disillusion which it breeds'; decentralise operational responsibility to Districts including some local responsibility for raising funds; and focus on quality and effectiveness as it was 'here that the NHS is in most danger'.[72] It was, they said, 'a period of economic difficulty and national political and social uncertainty'. The 1980s were to see the challenges for the NHS and Guy's and St Thomas' intensify significantly.

CHAPTER FOUR

Challenges and Changes, 1980-1991

Overview

The 1980s was a transformative decade for Guy's and St Thomas against a context of increasing financial pressures and the introduction of business models for the management, administration, and delivery of health services. The relationship between the hospitals and their local communities continued to evolve through the new health district structures. In response to wider initiatives to streamline medical and nursing training across London, including the Flowers' review of medical education, the merger of Guy's and St Thomas' medical schools was followed a few years later by that of the nursing schools. Both institutions continued to break new ground with Guy's successfully pioneering the introduction of the clinical directorate model to the UK and St Thomas' deepening public engagement with the heritage of the institution through the establishment of the Florence Nightingale Trust in 1982, leading to the opening of the Florence Nightingale Museum in 1989. The chapter ends with an account of the hospitals becoming NHS Trusts through the reforms introduced in the White Paper, *Working for Patients*.

Structural transformations

In April 1982, following the Health Services Act of 1980, the NHS was reorganised once again — the second time since its founding.

The area health authorities and district management teams introduced in the 1974 NHS reorganisation were replaced by 192 more localised district health authorities (DHAs). These DHAs were brought under the direction of the pre-existing regional health authorities (RHAs), which remained in place. The aims of the Thatcher Government's wide-reaching reforms were to: decentralise public health administration; devolve the decision-making process; and streamline services to alleviate the increasing financial burden of healthcare.[1] As Chapter 3 showed, the financial pressures had led to the Government appointing commissioners to run Lambeth, Southwark, and Lewisham AHA which had become 'unmanageable because it wouldn't work to a budget,' recalled Professor Malcom Forsythe, the Regional Medical Officer for the South East Region, 1978-92.[2] As smaller entities, DHAs would be closer to their local populations and so better able to assess local health needs, employ staff, and plan and administer hospital and community services under RHA guidance. The Act had a decisive impact on the NHS's administration, management and services. Following on so swiftly after the 1974 reorganisation, it set the pattern of continuous reform through reorganisation for the following decades.

Guy's and St Thomas' remained under the South East Thames RHA, but both fell under new respective DHAs. Guy's, formerly under the Guy's Health District (Teaching), was now within the Lewisham and North Southwark DHA; St Thomas', formerly under the St Thomas Health District (Teaching), now fell under the West Lambeth DHA. Amid the broader context of increasing financial pressures, the new system was characterised by tensions between the regional and district authorities. DHAs were expected to address local health needs through administering hospital and community services and employing staff. RHAs were distanced from day-to-day operations but continued to manage RAWP distributions and financing of specialist services across the region. Interviewees recounted the contentiousness of relationships between the DHAs and the RHA.

The first meeting of the West Lambeth DHA took place on 5 April 1982 although it had been meeting since autumn 1981 'in shadow'. The Chairman, Nick Cowan, with a background in personnel and industrial relations, described the Authority's 'biggest problem and the greatest challenge' as working within cash allocations: 'if we were to continue at present levels of activity we should need somewhere between £1m and £1.25m more than the total cash being made available to us this year...it is unrealistic to think that we shall be able to find the savings we need without painful changes. Practices that have existed for many years will have to end, many worthwhile aspirations will probably have to remain unfilled, activities undoubtedly worthwhile when considered solely in isolation will have to be curtailed'.[3] Five of the 13 members of the DHA were female but there were no members with an ethnically diverse background.[4]

Dr Stephen Jenkins chaired the District Management Team for West Lambeth DHA from 1984-86, served as District General Manager between 1987-89, and became Chief Executive Officer from 1989-90. 'My management career', Stephen recollects, 'started when I was appointed...as the Deputy Chairman of the District Management Team...I was in charge of valeting and car parking [at St Thomas'] and I'm happy to say I have no recollection about doing anything about either of those.' Looking back, Stephen felt that when he joined West Lambeth, things were governed more or less by 'consensus and bureaucracy'. St Thomas' had more than 107 committees alone. The relationship between the West Lambeth DHA and the RHA was fractious: 'the first half hour of any DHA budget meeting was trying to work out what fictions we told the RHA last year... The next part was spent on cooking up some more fictions for this year, and the third part, a brief assessment of how difficult it would be to support those fictions next year'.[5]

Along with many others working in Guy's or St Thomas' at the time, Stephen also recalled major political tensions that arose from the presence of hardline Labour councillors and union members within local government and the health authorities. Additional funding was available through joint finance initiatives with local authorities, but the ideological conflicts that had emerged in the late 1970s between the left-wing agendas of these local authorities and central government continued to play out in local resource allocation and made signing off on budgets virtually impossible. As Stephen noted: 'I found there were multiple agendas. I had West Lambeth District Health Authority, which was actually a sub-branch of Lambeth Council. It was diametrically opposed to anything that the then Government approved of. Entertainingly, it rarely ever set a budget for any given year. It had a very strong community bias, appropriately and rightly.'[6]

Led by Trotskyist Labour Councillor Ted Knight, Lambeth's local authorities during the period were increasingly seen as a 'hotbed' of radical leftism.[7] Hostile to the Thatcher Government and extremely cantankerous when it came to agreeing on the allocation of DHA resources, it took an overtly community-oriented approach, which often ran counter to the broader agenda of the RHA and its attempts to implement government policy. As Malcolm Forsythe who was Regional Medical Officer for the South East RHA during that period remembered: 'We had Ted Knight as one of our members and his technique was to keep adjourning meetings, so they just never progressed. It was actually very difficult trying to run the show with the union and local authority representation on the area health authorities and the region.'[8] For people like Patricia Moberly who had worked through the earlier and more collegiate periods of the Lambeth, Southwark, and Lewisham AHA, the changes were 'really rather tragic'.[9]

Nor were Guy's experiences of the Lewisham and North Southwark DHA any smoother. Elaine Murphy had trained at Manchester

Medical School and specialised in psychiatry. She joined Guy's in 1983 as its first female professor and became District General Manager in the same year: 'Of my 24 or so health authority members,' she said, 'about three quarters of them were, frankly, left, very far left, as they were on Lewisham council and Southwark council. And so, steering a course, for example, on competitive tendering was a nightmare; a nightmare.'[10] The intention that the new structures would streamline decision-making and deliver budget-setting and resource allocation was thus thwarted by local and political disputes.

Furthermore, 1982 saw strong union resistance to decreases in NHS expenditure under the Thatcher Government, which culminated in industrial action. In April, 13 unions demanded a 12 per cent pay increase for health service workers, rejecting a divisive offer of a 6.4 per cent to nurses and four per cent to other workers. The dispute encompassed nurses, nursing auxiliaries, porters, cleaners, and other non-medical staff; however, nurses stuck to the Royal College of Nurses' (RCN) long-standing policy that they would not strike. According to the West Lambeth DHA's magazine, *Circle*, union action restricted admissions to Accident and Emergency at St Thomas', reduced daily operations by 60 per cent, six wards closed, and the outpatients' ambulance service was affected which infringed the TUC Code of Conduct. The correspondent reflected on the changing nature of the dispute, with the Central Sterile Supplies Department strike causing shortages of sterile equipment between June and August, with a picket line subsequently set up by the Shop Steward's Committee. The *Circle* speculated: 'at times during the action concern has been expressed that the hospital might close'.[11] The Government stood firm and NHS historian Geoffrey Rivett noted that union tactics 'turned the press and public and drove a wedge between them and the RCN'.[12] In December 1982, the unions settled for a lower pay offer over two years with nurses offered their own independent pay review body, announced in July 1983. But the settlement was to be short-lived, with many continuing to feel the reduction in wages in real terms.

Lee Soden joined Guy's in 1978 as the District Catering Manager and remembered the ways catering staff worked discreetly to ensure patients did not suffer from the industrial action whilst also avoiding confrontation with the unions. But he also suffered damage to his car after delivering milk to St Olave's Hospital which had many elderly patients at the time:

> I used to have a beautiful blue Triumph Spitfire, wonderful car, with a Californian top and it was my pride and joy, and I was delivering milk to St Olave's one day…because they weren't going to let milk in…it was an elderly care facility at the time and the union down there was particularly strong… I was just about to sell this car and the following night, having delivered the milk, there was £400 worth of damage done to my car…Would I do the same again? Yes, I would because the people in bed couldn't do anything about it.

One of the positive outcomes of the strikes were that practices changed 'because management had to get their hands dirty and work and understand what it was really about, and it was good'.[13]

In London many smaller hospitals had closed or been amalgamated with larger ones through the 1960s and 1970s. In the 1980s the reforms to the larger London hospitals including Guy's and St Thomas' were strongly resisted amidst wider concerns about the privatisation of the NHS. As in Lambeth and Southwark, Labour-led local authorities opposed national Conservative policies and in 1983 the London Health Emergency group was formed forging an alliance of campaigners against hospital closures and by extension included unions representing various occupations in the NHS.[14] The umbrella group was initially funded by Greater London Council (GLC), led by Ken Livingstone.

Mergers

It was a period when broader questions were being raised about the interface between the NHS and the universities and their respective function and responsibilities for care of patients, and undergraduate and postgraduate education in biomedical, clinical, and health services research. The climate of financial stringency added sharpness to the discussions.[15]

Frederick Dainton had established the first new medical school of the twentieth century in Nottingham and chaired a government inquiry into the declining numbers of students studying science and technology in universities. He argued that DHAs which had oversight of teaching hospitals needed a better appreciation of the contribution these hospitals made to the NHS because this provided the context for decision-making and resource allocation.[16]

> A District Health Authority which manages university hospitals is the place where the future confronts the present and the problem is to make this confrontation productive rather than cause sterile and destructive tensions.[17]

With hindsight it is clear how these debates foreshadowed the later development of Academic Health Sciences Centres. Alongside the structural transformation of the NHS, Guy's and St Thomas' and their neighbouring institutions were affected by medical education reforms. In 1980, *London Medical Education – a New Framework* was published as the report of a working party on medical and dental teaching resources chaired by Brian Hilton Flowers (Baron Flowers FRS), Rector of Imperial College London.[18] The Flowers Review addressed London's sprawling medical educational provision, which remained intact despite the recommendations of Lord Todd in 1968 that the overprovision should be addressed through mergers.[19] Flowers recommended that London's 33 medical and dental education institutions should be consolidated into just six. Whereas Todd's review in 1968 had proposed pairing Guy's Hospital Medical School with King's College Hospital Medical School and St Thomas' Hospital Medical School with St George's Hospital Medical School, Flowers' Review went much further: the medical schools of Guy's, St Thomas' and Kings College should all amalgamate under the banner of 'Lister and St Thomas'.[20] The suggestion that Guy's and King's would relinquish the histories embedded in their names was abhorrent and indeed, the continued use of St Thomas' in the banner only intensified the depth of rivalries between the institutions. As noted previously, mergers were highly problematic because the continuity of each institution's history was embedded in its specific name, which became core to the identity of students and staff and emblematic of the respective culture.

Tim Matthews, later Chief Executive Officer at St Thomas', began his career as an administration trainee for the Civil Service, working on the Flowers Review amongst other Department of Health and Social Services reviews. Tim reflects on the negative effects of the dispersal of clinical specialisms across many hospitals that informed Flowers' recommendations.

> There had been a growing sense, for some time, that London's hospitals had great reputations, had great clinicians, had good research, but a lot of their departments were too small, so the research and clinical excellence was spread too thin, so there was a good deal of pressure to look at ways in which departments might be amalgamated, but, of course, that meant hospitals giving up some services and almost trading some services for another. And, you know, what became very apparent very early on, and I was quite

a junior official at that time, was that tribal loyalty was as strong an emotive in a lot of hospitals as achieving clinical or research excellence.[21]

Tim Clark trained at Guy's in the 1950s and worked at the Hammersmith Hospital before returning as a senior lecturer in physiology and medicine with an honorary senior registrar appointment to the hospital. His period away from Guy's had given him a perspective that made him very concerned about the future.

> I didn't think Guy's had a future much longer, or Thomas', of just being dependent on part time consultant surgeons and physicians, who spent a lot of time in Harley Street. Who were very good doctors and very good teachers of medicine, but that was it. So the view I came back to Guy's with was not unique to me. There was quite a lot of concern at the time that Guy's would never become famous again. There was a feeling that the future was not continuing in the way of the past. It did need to embrace the academic side of things, and that meant embracing up to then [what had been] a non-entity, the University of London.

By the time the Flowers Review was published, Tim had just become dean-elect and remembers the Review sparking questions about: how are we going to survive as a hospital?[22]

Consolidating London's medical education establishments was one facet of civil service recommendations focussed on the capital. The non-executive London Health Planning Consortium (LHPC), founded in 1977 and chaired by John Smith, a DHSS officer (also chair of the earlier RAWP), identified the over-concentration of acute services in London as the population living in the inner parts of the capital decreased. The LHPC's report on the reconfiguration of hospitals – *Towards a balance* – was published alongside Flowers' review in 1980. In response to the changing demographic patterns, it proposed that teaching hospitals in central London should form relationships with large hospitals further out of the metropolis to better meet the changing patient inflows and outflows.[23]

In anticipation of the upheavals in medical education, St Thomas' had taken the decision at the Leeds Castle workshop in 1979 that it would be better to approach Guy's with a view to merging medical schools than wait for change to be imposed, as recounted in Chapter 3. Gastroenterologist Brian Creamer had become Dean of St Thomas' Medical School in 1979 and within a week of taking up the post he was visited by Lord Flowers, 'outlining his plan for closing our preclinical school to put it in King's'. It was a 'shock tactic' that was replicated across London, reflected Brian. Guy's was the obvious partner: 'we were close, we thought the same and the solution seemed right.'[24] The merger took place in 1982 and established the United Medical Schools of Guy's and St Thomas' with Tim Clark as Dean; 1983 heralded further amalgamations when the United Medical Schools of Guy's and St Thomas' integrated the Royal Dental Hospital of London School of Dental Surgery which 'strengthened considerably the research of the combined school' and formed the United Medical and Dental Schools of Guy's and St Thomas' (UMDS).[25] In 1985, the Postgraduate Institute of Dermatology came on board.

The difficulties of merging teaching schools played out in dentistry as well as medicine. The proposals, reflected Ian Gainsford, Dean of King's College Hospital Dental School from 1977 to 1987, were 'totally unsatisfactory' in terms of teaching whole-mouth patient care.

> What they forgot to recognise was that both at Guy's Hospital and at King's College Hospital there was a dental school as well as medical schools and no thought had been given as to how to merge the two. One couldn't have part

of the dental course taught at Guy's and part of the dental course taught at King's. One had to recognise, in teaching students, you had to treat patients as a whole. You couldn't say, 'This patient A needs a denture and needs a filling in a tooth by the side of the denture; we'll send the patient to Guy's for the filling and send the patient to King's for the denture'; I mean it becomes a nonsense for the patient. The treatment plan had to be geared to the interests of the patient, not only to the interests of training the student. They had added a rider, which was obviously a nonsense, that in the event of the merging of Guy's and King's Dental School on the Guy's site, they would think in terms of closing the dental school at King's and building a new dental school at possibly St Mary's, but that really was a non-starter; the sheer costs of doing that was crazy and so of course it became a major issue. We in fact won the day by King's College Dental School remaining. In fact, it was University College Dental School that closed. This was a pity because 'as the pendulum swings' there arose a shortage of dentists requiring the Government to inject a huge sum of money to re-establish a new dental school.[26]

Though the merger was accepted as the 'right' solution and one which enabled the institutions in Brian's words to restructure 'on our own terms', the impact was felt by many to be sudden and enormous.[27] It 'came as a bombshell', remarked Barry Jackson, who became a governor at UMDS from 1989 to 1994. Though trained at King's College, London, Barry was a consultant surgeon at St Thomas', which he describes with warmth. He also expressed 'huge affection' for his colleagues at Guy's and ultimately believed the merging of medical schools was for the best. 'When it came, I supported it,' he said, whilst acknowledging the different opinions across both institutions.[28] Richard Thompson, lead consultant of endoscopy at St Thomas', saw the strengths of each teaching style with St Thomas' 'concentrated on clinical medicine…Guy's was much more academically orientated, so in a sense joining with them brought those two things together'. Richard describes the strength of feeling at the time and explains how he believed the institutional alliance played out.

> Brian Creamer was the [St Thomas'] Dean then, and he, like me, I think was very sad of the idea of a merger, but he realised that…the only way to save it was to be United Medical School of Guy's and Thomas'…by fusing the ones. He got hold of the Dean there, who was George Houston I think…and he obviously made a plan to save the medical schools by the two fusing together, otherwise I think we wouldn't have closed the hospital, we'd have lost the medical school, which would have been a great sadness.[29]

The merger was promoted as a collegiate arrangement similar to Oxbridge: 'that always made everyone purr, oh, good, like Oxbridge, that's fine. We will have Guy's and Thomas' which, rather like Oxbridge colleges, will retain their separate identities and personality, but we will have a merged administration. Nobody ever minded what happened to administration, which was a highly pejorative word,' reflected Ian Cameron, Dean of UMDS between 1986 and 1989.[30] Writing in 1986, Brian Creamer explained that although UMDS were now introducing a single prospectus and a single entry system, because UMDS had 'won' the right to keep the 'collegiate identities' of the two medical schools, prospective students would be offered the choice of Guy's or St Thomas' as UMDS was a 'two college institution with all the advantages that brings'.[31]

The slow pace of change helped people adapt to a new status quo.

> The UMDS merger happened very subtly. We were UMDS for many years before anybody realised that their medical

school had gone, because the students were either taught on the St Thomas' site or the Guy's site, and all we did was to actually coalesce, or make our syllabus identical so we all taught the same thing. And then at the end of the day when they applied for house jobs you could apply for a house job anywhere, and so some of the Guy's graduates went and worked at Thomas' and some of the Thomas' people came to work at Guy's. We worked relatively happily alongside our colleagues on the education committees to deliver a reasonable curriculum. So that did work quite well.[32]

Elaine Murphy had joined Guy's as professor of psychiatry in the year of the merger.

I couldn't really see anything going on. I knew that there had been resistance, and I knew there was tremendous anxiety…I knew that there was great jockeying for position and that…working out the administrative team support from the administrators of the universities was difficult. I knew that the people who were running it were sort of tearing out their hair…But as a junior professor, you know, a brand new professor, I was really focusing on what I'd gone there to do, which was develop the service and, you know, try to get psychiatry of old age looked on as something completely different and something that could generate prestige teams, and that we were doing something valuable for the local community and that it was a thing you could attract good people into… So, I was very, very busy and didn't really notice what was going on, you know, at UMDS…I mean, during my time, I only ever taught Guy's students. Then finally, I think in my last two to three years, somebody said, oh, you're a professor of UMDS, would you like to do a lecture every now and again at Thomas'? But, you know, it was actually down the river, you know, it was a long way away, we thought it was a long way away. And it was a long walk, it was quicker by boat…they were deciding to join up the degrees and the student entry when I left, I think. And that was not long before they started all the discussions with King's that went on for years and years.[33]

Hywel Thomas, a tutor in biochemistry, recalled the gradual logistical changes resulting from the merger.

We started moving departments around about mid/late 1980s, moving anatomy to Guy's, physiology to Thomas' initially, two big moves needing a lot of work to be done: building new dissecting rooms and laboratories, computer laboratories, things of this kind. Students had to move between the campuses, but we took care that they never had to move during the day, they would spend one, two days St Thomas', three at Guy's or vice versa.[34]

Disruption to established working patterns was an inevitable consequence of such changes. At Guy's, for example, some dental teaching staff were actively involved in physiological research and the move of the physiology department to a different site made it more difficult to integrate research into working patterns. Nevertheless, the Dental School accepted the changes were in the best interests of UMDS. Stephen Challacombe trained in dentistry at Guy's and at the time of the mergers was on the Council of the Medical School. He was very involved in the merger discussions.

These were managed pretty well, given that they were two proud medical schools merging. I think there was a sense of balance and fairness very early on, which was not repeated when we came to the hospital side, but a sense of balance where, for instance, anatomy was to be taught on one site and physiology on another, that pharmacology would be taught on the Guy's site and biochemistry...or vice versa actually, at St Thomas'. So, there's a sense of balance and we...gradually realised that by pulling in the same direction, that actually there were going to be great strengths from merging the schools.[35]

Running Guy's and St Thomas' medical schools along separate lines under one overarching joint administration was a pragmatic response to the practical and emotional consequences of mergers. The strength of institutional loyalty amongst students and staff was immense and they had a 'homing instinct to their alma mater', noted Jangu Banatvala who joined St Thomas' in 1965 to set up a virology department.[36] Ian Gainsford explains that previously, 'when a medical student or a dental student went to, say Guy's, all his time as a student was spent at Guy's; he didn't associate at all with students of other faculties, he would be totally encompassed within the hospital environment, he would be a St Thomas' student or a Guy's student'.[37] It took until the 1989-1990 academic year for the first 'truly' UMDS cohort to be taught their preclinical subjects equally between the Guy's and St Thomas' campuses.

The UMDS merger also signalled broader changes to the style of medical education which weakened the strong historical ties between the students and teaching institutions. A consultant at St Thomas' reflected on the shift in his memoir.

> The students at that time had a close attachment to the wards, had a caseload of their own patients who they were expected to see every day and accompany to the theatre or X-ray or wherever, which taught them to empathise and understand what it was like to be a patient and to develop a sense of responsibility. Now they sit in lecture theatres for much of the time and when they appear on the wards

or outpatient departments their primary intention is to get their 'book' signed up. They have no allegiance it seems to a team, a group of patients, even to a hospital.[38]

One of the most fraught areas was the integration of the student bodies of the two schools, particularly sports clubs. Writing in the West Lambeth Health Authority District magazine in 1990, Ian Cameron, Dean of UMDS between 1986 and 1989 noted: 'We have now achieved, after some knife-edge diplomacy, union of the Students Clubs with a new, agreed constitution.'[39] David Barlow, who trained at St Thomas' and became a consultant in genitourinary medicine, was invited to be a St Thomas' representative on the committee for the amalgamation. Working with a Guy's physician 'the two of us had to try and smooth over the waters'.[40] In many personal recollections from students and staff of both hospitals, cultural differences were most starkly expressed in the context of sports. Merging the boat clubs was one of the most fraught activities. David noted that: 'we used to win or come very close to the head of the river race. Whereas Guy's was probably a more all-encompassing club, and in that respect a better club because anybody could join. But there was a great antagonism…it was a difficult time when the two medical schools joined together'.[41] In spring 1989 Matthew Solan, St Thomas' Rugby Club Captain wrote: 'The end of an era – RIP St Thomas' RFC.' It was 'very sad', he continued, for anyone who respects the 'proud traditions of the hospital's history,' but added that 'it is important to start the new era with the same enthusiasm that made the last 125 years so successful'.[42] But the differences across sports translated into broader culture clashes as Jangu Banatvala, then President of the St Thomas' boat club, explained.

I suppose Guy's were sharper in some ways, very good physicians, good surgeons particularly, and we were a little more gentlemanly perhaps in our approach. You saw that with the students at first [after the UMDS merger] and then as time went on there was no difference. I felt 'Thomas' students knew how to dress properly for a party and how to tie a bow tie. I'm not so sure some of the Guy's did... the merger of the boat clubs caused more problems than anything else I think, which we eventually achieved. Of course, they said, well, with the merger of the boat clubs... we will win every event at Henley. Of course, they got worse in fact.[43]

As for previous generations of students, the bar remained a hub for meeting people. Tony Gardner trained at Guy's in the early 1980s.

Guy's bar was renowned throughout the country for being the cheapest bar in London. The students ran it until they realised, they were losing so much money, not through anyone embezzling, just because they were useless, so they got a barman in. It was a meeting point for medical students, dental students, physiotherapists, nurses, radiographers. And not everyone liked it, but it became your hub. This is in the days before mobile phones. We couldn't text or phone each other. The bar would open at five and we'd know that if you went down at seven o'clock on a Friday or after sport on a Wednesday everyone would be there.[44]

Medical students had a long history of rowdy behaviour but during the 1980s as social attitudes towards race and gender were changing, medical student culture was increasingly viewed as deeply offensive. In 1984 the Guy's *Wag Mag* was the subject of a critical editorial in the *Sunday Observer* newspaper. It contains 'some of the most tasteless jokes ... they are racist, offensive, rude, and unfunny' it noted.[45] Further public criticism came from Labour MP Terry Davis who noted that Guy's should be training doctors whose ideas of humanity were aligned to a multi-racial society.[46]

Clinicians and management

One of the most significant changes of the 1980s for the hospitals was the introduction of general management following the 1983 inquiry into NHS management under the chairmanship of Roy Griffiths, Managing Director of J Sainsbury plc.[47] Peter Griffiths, the District Administrator and District General Manager for the Lewisham and North Southwark Health Authority between 1982 and 1989 recalls how the report led to the appointment of general managers across the NHS.

> Roy Griffiths was the managing director of Sainsbury's at the time and had been invited by the Conservative Government to review manpower in the NHS but came up with a report that actually reviewed the management of the NHS and suggested that the health service was short of the equivalent of chief executives and running on a consensus management system was not appropriate in his view. So, I became District General Manager of Lewisham and North Southwark Health Authority having been its district administrator.[48]

In earlier decades when resources were more plentiful, relationships between senior doctors, nurses, and administrators in both institutions had been good. But dissatisfaction about the funding decisions taken by administrators in the context of cash limits had been building since the late 1970s. At Guy's Hospital, Cyril Chantler had battled to secure the resources needed for the paediatric renal unit to the extent of making the issues public by being filmed standing by an empty cot and explaining he needed more nurses to support the service.

> Guy's was in chaos, beds were being cut, the doctors and the administration weren't really engaged with each other, we were constantly having debates in television studios, which

should have been taking place in the hospital. I remember an administrator saying to me one night, he said, Cyril, if you'd stop admitting patients to this hospital, I'd have no trouble running it...the film was shown to Ken Clarke, then Secretary of State for Health who commented, if he'd start doing what Guy's wants him to do, rather than what he wants to do, maybe we would all be a bit happier![49]

Matters came to a crunch in January 1984 when the District Management Team decided to close more than 100 beds and over the following two months increased demand for services led Guy's to become 'the first London hospital to spend more money by closing beds'.[50] Cyril was one of a small group of clinicians who had been observing the introduction of decentralised management structures at Johns Hopkins Hospital in Baltimore, US. The District Management Team was 'persuaded' to visit to see at first-hand how such a management structure might work. In the autumn of 1984, Guy's Medical and Dental Committee voted to establish a new hospital management board which would take over the running of the hospital in April 1985. The change required clinicians to adopt a new mindset that broadened their responsibilities for patient care from individual to population level.

> With my colleagues I argued that clinicians in a publicly funded healthcare system needed to accept that profligacy in the care of one patient could lead to the denial of adequate care to another. It therefore becomes an ethical responsibility to encourage efficacy, effectiveness, efficiency, equity, economy, and excellence of quality.[51]

Jeremy Brinley Codd who had joined Guy's in 1980 to work in the finance department affirmed that the clinical budgeting initiative was driven by clinicians, 'there was a great thirst for it, there were a lot of very senior, well-respected clinicians in the hospital and there was a great willingness and desire to do this'.[52] Under the new arrangements, clinicians would take full responsibility for the operational management of the hospital including financial accountability, in return for the authority to influence the allocation of resources. The team accepted a revenue reduction of £8 million per year over three years which amounted to a reduction of around 15 per cent per year. The challenges were enormous as the capital expenditure needs had been stockpiled, including repairing the cooling system in Guy's Tower, installing a new air-conditioning system for the operating theatres and much more repair and upgrading work.[53] Clinical directorates were established and budgets were decentralised to directorate level and included staff costs (clinical and ancillary), drugs, maintenance of equipment, investigations, and eventually the use of additional services such as intensive care and/or operating theatres. At the end of the initial three-year period 'both the quality and the quantity of patients' care' was preserved.[54] Cyril's personal commitment to the initiative and his outstanding ability to motivate people to work to a common cause through chairing the Management Board led to its eventual success. He reflected that 'what was most impressive was the changing and improved relationship between different health professionals and administrators'.[55]

St Thomas' had a solid history of adopting business approaches to management as described in Chapter 2 under the leadership of John Wyn Owen. Staff awareness of costs and the need for efficiency was widespread. In 1980 Maureen Dillon, Superintendent Physiotherapist, came up with the idea of holding exhibitions entitled *What it Costs* to help staff become: 'more aware of what things cost, we can help to prevent waste and get the best value for money within the District'. The first exhibition focused on physiotherapy, showcasing the cost of a wheelchair at almost £200 and a Zimmer Frame at £14. The second was themed on the costs of the day-to-day running of offices across the District, and included facts such as the quarterly telephone bill amounted to £32,000 and the cost of a bleep was £170. Costs for the Domestic Department were £4 million a year and 90 per cent of that money was used for staff labour costs.[56] Following the Griffiths Report, involvement of clinicians in management was also adopted at St Thomas'. Initial resistance came from the '2000 club', founded by a group of young consultants who anticipated working in the hospital in the year 2000. Their aim was to challenge the concept of 'clinical management', yet they were invited to become involved with the changes.

> We must have been taken seriously because several of us were shortly afterwards invited to a meeting with the 'management' of the hospital and asked how we would arrange for clinicians to be embedded in the management process. We devised an Executive Management Team for the hospital that allocated the clinical specialties into five different areas each led by a clinician, then there would be five non-doctor managers (one of whom was the Head Nurse, ie Matron) and of course also the Chief Executive. Doctors, if supported by Matron, therefore retained a power of veto. We and surprisingly they, were happy with that and the Executive Management Team was set up. It included four of the 2000 Club. The Chief Executive…was in fact a clinician, a cardiologist, but was judged ineffective as a Chief Executive so we doctors quickly began plotting to remove him.[57]

Another member recollected:

> I wish I'd kept the back of the envelope on which we first designed the management executive of Thomas', which, if I remember it, was an A4 envelope, third of A4, and we drew a little table on it, and down one side we put the managers that would have to be the finance manager, the

chief executive and so on down one side that would have to be on the board, and then we made up enough clinical sub-groups for the other side so that we would have the same number of sort of voters on either side of the table. That worked fine.[58]

Nevertheless, the new management processes did not protect St Thomas' from further financial crisis in October 1987 when savings of £2.5 million needed to be made to keep within cash limits. A wide range of options had been proposed to the West Lambeth DHA from redesignating 16 beds for use by private patients which would have produced savings of £727,000 over a full year, to reducing the carpentry service to essential maintenance only resulting in savings of £30,000.[59] The most high-profile measure was the closure of 137 beds for a period of months. Nurses voiced their concern about the effects on patient care through a 'bed push' of 137 beds across Westminster Bridge and a week-long vigil outside Parliament during which nurses and students wore black armbands to 'mourn' the beds. John Garnett, Chairman of the West Lambeth DHA, had made the case to the Department of Health for more money, but the staff magazine also called for 'everyone's help and ideas. These could include selling of services, identifying new sources of income, or anything else you may think of, no matter how "way out"'.[60] The matter was hotly disputed in debates in the House of Commons. Stuart Holland, Labour MP for Vauxhall, highlighted the difficulties that resulted from St Thomas' drawing most of its patients from outside the district. The bed use rate was running at 98.5 per cent and the waiting list stood at over two thousand patients. There were no more savings, he said, to be made from cutting support or ancillary services. St Thomas' consultants were so appalled by the situation that they had offered to contribute five per cent from their salaries as a short-term measure. The reply from Edwina Currie, then Parliamentary Under-Secretary for Health and Social Security, was robust: 'Whatever difficulties are currently being experienced must be set against that background of growth, expansion, and excellence. Any Hon Member would give their eye teeth to have a hospital of the quality of St Thomas's in their constituency.'[61]

By 1987 Guy's had undergone its programme of rationalisation that included cuts and redundancies and was in a more stable financial position. Witnessing the events at St Thomas', a senior registrar from the renal unit who had strongly opposed the Guy's strategy took time to write to Cyril Chantler to apologise for his earlier stance on the issue.

> I came across a letter addressed to you, written by me at the end of 1985…I think it may have been provoked by…a second batch of redundancies at Guy's. On re-reading the letter, almost two years later, and with the benefit of hindsight, I would certainly wish to change a substantial proportion of it…Your strategy was to implement a rationalisation programme involving some cuts but preserving the core activities at Guy's' and safeguarding capital development. My strategy, at the time as I recall it, was one of obstructionism. Having witnessed the cuts that have proved necessary at some of neighbouring hospitals where the cuts have been late and consequently more savage, I must confess you have been vindicated by events. I am particularly convinced by our sister hospital, St Thomas', where it seems the plan is to reduce it to half the size of a district general hospital. By these standards, the cutbacks that occurred in Guy's in 1984-5 seem relatively minor.[62]

From the Department of Health and Social Security's perspective, the political lobbying from the hospitals on matters of funding was intense and impossible to escape during this period, reflected Dr

Graham Winyard who joined the Department as Senior Principal
Medical Officer in 1987.

> One of the elements in the mix, it felt to me, was hospitals
> such as Guy's were lobbying passionately about the fact that
> the system, as it then was, punished centres of excellence
> that could attract lots of patients – that the money did not
> flow with the patients, and this was seen by them as an
> outrage. They seemed to be quite well-connected in to the
> Prime Minister in ways I never fully understood, but you
> felt that Ian McColl [Professor of Surgery at Guy's] could
> bend ears. From day one, it felt that the Department was
> under siege, with each day bringing new stories of service
> shortcomings which regional liaison and its medical group
> had to devise responses to.[63]

Jeremy Brinley Codd who worked in Guy's finance department at
the time affirms that political lobbying was part of everyday life.

> Well, I remember one of the clinical directors of surgery
> at Guy's saying to me one afternoon, Jeremy, how much
> money do we need, I'm having tea with Margaret Thatcher
> this afternoon! And he was advisor to Margaret Thatcher
> and, after that, to John Major on health and that was
> Professor Lord McColl, a well-known surgeon, and so there
> was great political play going on behind the scenes. At that
> stage, I wasn't any part of that at all.[64]

Changes to nursing

As in medicine and dentistry, national changes to the education
and training of nurses during the 1980s disrupted long-established
patterns of practice in the institutions' nursing schools. Since the
nineteenth century, student nurses had been trained on the wards

and were inculcated in the specific practices and cultures of each hospital. Nurses were as devoted to their institution as doctors. Since the early years of the NHS, two parallel training routes had been offered: the State Enrolled Nurse (SEN) certificate and the State Registered Nurse (SRN) certificate.[65] It was the SRN that provided the more rigorous qualification, with the two-year SEN qualification offering little mobility across the profession. This two-tier system of educating nurses, both hospital care orientated, reinforced wider social inequalities arising from race and class. The SRN was an established route into nursing for white, middle-class women, whilst nursing recruits from overseas or ethnically diverse backgrounds were channelled into the SEN training, 'frequently and deliberately'.[66] The distinctions made between the two types of training affected nurses' prospects for accreditation and promotion in the hospitals. Eddyna Danso was born in Sierra Leone and her family moved to England in the 1960s. Her first job on leaving school was as a lab assistant in a pharmaceutical company but the low rates of pay led her to look for new opportunities and she joined Guy's Hospital to train as a theatre technician in 1973. She reflected on Black nurses' experiences of the different nurse training schemes.

Those cousins and relatives I was talking to, even though they had 'A' levels and so on, came here and they had to do the SEN course first, because that's what they were advised to do. And then, later on, when they became more aware, they went on to do their SRN. So, you find that the Black nurses were over-qualified...so they'll do three years for their SEN, then maybe another two years to do their SRN, then maybe another two years to do their midwifery, or if they wanted to do mental nursing, or community, health visitors as it was called, any speciality. So, you know, when you've got that situation where the first advice you're given, and because you've come abroad, you don't want to start arguing. And the way we were brought up back home,

you know, you had deference, you had respect for people,
for authority, if they say, okay, I think the SEN course is
good for you, then, you know, they accepted it, until when,
as they became wise, they then, you know, went on to do
different. But it was very hard.[67]

In 1986 the Central Council for Nursing and Midwifery (UKCC)
published their reform agenda: *Project 2000: a new preparation for
practice*, which would remove the two-tier system with the creation
of a three-year Registered Nursing certificate. It also marked the
movement of nursing education from hospitals to higher education,
reflecting the shift to wider nursing needs in the community and
for mental health support, where rigid ward practice was not useful
preparation.[68] The central aim of *Project 2000* was to change the over-
reliance upon students in the workforce, a recurrent theme in every
proposal on nursing reform since the 1940s. *Project 2000* also aimed to
reduce the high turnover of nurses, which during training was seven
to 20 per cent, with a further 15 to 20 per cent failing exams.[69]

Discussions in Guy's Hospital magazine, *Guylines*, reveal how
nursing hierarchies appeared unwelcoming for nursing students.
In 1981, K Oxley, a student nurse wrote 'when I emerged onto the
ward for the first time it was disappointing to find the qualified staff
not as approachable as I had anticipated. It seemed that ease of
communication depended on the colour of one's belt, which in turn
was a sign of one's experience and knowledge'. Frances Jones, a sister
on Charles Symonds Ward, responded to criticisms, suggesting that:
'what Nurse Oxley and others who feel like her fail to realise is that it
is worth enduring all the hardships of student nurse training in order
to qualify and to have the satisfaction of changing things… Attitudes
have changed quite dramatically since I qualified seven years ago and,
hopefully, will continue to change'.[70] The divisive nature of internal
hierarchies, even between different year groups of nursing students,
was one of the problems identified as a factor in the loss of nurses

in a 1985 Commission on Nursing Education chaired by Dr Henry Judge.[71] *Project 2000* also advocated grants for student nurses, and a conversion course to bring SEN staff up to the SRN level. Eddyna Danso, discussing the plight of her colleagues from Black and ethnic minority backgrounds, noted that the conversion course was free of charge at Guy's and St Thomas' and King's College: 'a lot of nurses who were qualified from abroad took advantage of that, whilst I know in other hospitals, they had to pay for it or, you know, they funded it themselves'.[72]

Just as in the medical schools, nursing schools built strong institutional relationships with their students, which meant that staff who qualified elsewhere could find it difficult to integrate. One interviewee who described training at Lewisham Hospital in the 1960s when the strict nursing hierarchies left students 'running scared' of their seniors joined the Nightingale School in 1982. It was, they said, an insular place: 'almost as though it was cocooned from the outside world and whatever happened out there wouldn't affect them, you know'. Religion and ethnicity were also factors and although they did not find their own progression negatively impacted by their Catholicism, other staff shared with them examples of discrimination against Irish or Catholic nurses which had limited their ability to progress upwards. They also recalled a senior staff member explaining that St Thomas' was shaped by other hidden networks including freemasonry.[73] Hywel Thomas, a biochemistry tutor, echoed these views.

> I think it was renowned as being very traditional, rather backward looking, archaic in many ways, snobby, I mentioned that it had to be said, that was a view for a long time, hierarchical, at one point, a lot of the establishment was dominated by the Masons, you know, they had a strong masonic streak running through it. What's happened these days to a lot of those things, I don't know, I think a lot

of that has melted away now, because it's had to join the modern world.[74]

The 1980s was a time of growing awareness of the barriers that could affect social opportunities, but nursing cultures remained firmly embedded in the past. In 1987 the Nightingale School of Nursing was found guilty of racial discrimination against a Black applicant for a tutor's job.[75] Graham Haynes had joined the Nightingale School of Nursing in 1985 as Nursing Tutor and found that social assumptions dictated admissions policy: 'I sat on interview panels and the director of nursing education looked at me and said, 'well, this one is easy, Daddy is a judge,' so that was an automatic entrance to nursing. The fact that the student probably had three legs and no brain had nothing to do with it!'[76] Patricia Moberly had continued her interest in health matters as a member of North Lewisham and Southwark DHA and she also taught English in Pimlico in a school which recruited large numbers of students from the Vauxhall area. The school was mixed but there were some 'very, very clever kids' who were fast-tracked for O'Level exams and took two subjects a year early. In their O'Level year these students would then commence A'Level studies and complete the remaining five O'Level exams.

> One of these very clever girls, who ended up with seven 'As', two of which she'd got early, applying for St Thomas', and being turned down without an interview for the nursing school. And I was absolutely furious, and I came storming over here, into this very building, because that was the nursing school, on the ground floor. Going to see the Director of Nursing and saying, you said, you wanted six good 'O' Levels and now I have a girl with seven 'A's and you have refused even to see her. "Well, she didn't get them all at the same time." I said, no, she didn't get them all at the same time, because if you looked at her application, you would have seen that she was so bright that I personally

entered her early for two of them. "Well, I'm sorry she didn't get them all at the same time, so we can't interview her." Savage!

This drove Patricia to visit the science inspector at County Hall and develop a pilot scheme to widen access to St Thomas' for children from the state sector. It was 'like pulling teeth' getting St Thomas' to consider it: "'Mrs Moberly, we can get nice girls from nice homes to this nursing school," said the Director of Nursing.'

> The concept that anyone in a London day school, a mere comprehensive, couldn't be a nice girl from a nice home, well, I was not happy at all. And I've always felt very strongly since then about proper access and proper fairness in recruitment. I mean, it's a different world now. That wouldn't happen, but the concept of diversity and transparency and fairness, simply didn't exist then. People didn't discuss it.[77]

As later chapters illustrate, Patricia continued her campaign to embed these values across Guy's and St Thomas' when she became Chairman in 1999.

The employment of ethnically diverse staff at Guy's and St Thomas' during this period began to increase and led to the hospitals' communities better reflecting the ethnicity of the local communities. For some patients and families, encounters with NHS staff provided the first opportunity for coming close to people with different ethnic backgrounds.

> Nurse Angie, for example, she was probably from an Indian, Pakistani background. So, there were things to adjust to that we were not used to, from having lived exclusively amongst white people in the UK in the '70s and '80s, but

which are now ubiquitous in society and, you know, sort of, it's not new, is it? But there had always to be people's first encounter from being, you know, a sort of almost all white community with the kind of multi-racial culture which was already in Central London. So, there were cultural aspects like that, that were different about Guy's.[78]

Patricia Mowbray who worked as Art Historian at St Thomas' between 1975 and 1986 remembered the first Black sister joining the hospital's Eye Department, in the early 1980s. It was also around that time that a group of Black midwives were appointed to the Midwifery Department in Block 8: 'they were wonderful women; I watched them holding newborn babies, cuddling them and sometimes crooning and I thought what a wonderful start for entry into a strange new life'.[79]

Strong professional identities aligned to specific institutions were created during nurse training, just as in medicine. At St Thomas' the historical links with Florence Nightingale were paramount in shaping nursing identities. Liz Jenkins, who trained at St Thomas' in the 1960s, noted that Nightingale nurses 'felt special' and in turn 'behaved specially'.[80] In practice, Nightingale nurses trained for a further year beyond their certificates and wore a badge to distinguish their expertise. Natalie Tiddy, a Nightingale nurse at St Thomas' who rose through management roles, explains:

> At the end of the three years, having passed the GNC, General Nursing Council examination, here at St Thomas' you did an extra year to get your Nightingale badge, so I worked for an extra year to get my Nightingale badge. It was what they called payback time. They'd trained us, now we give something back was the general idea. All of us had four- or three-month allocations in that last year, which we were placed into, you didn't have a choice. One of mine

was paediatrics, and one of mine was three months' night duty, and one of mine was Edward ward where I went on to become a senior staff nurse.[81]

Mike Messer, photographer at St Thomas', remembered nurses placing a posy of flowers in the hand of the statue of Florence Nightingale to mark her birthday every year. Her legacy stretched far beyond the wards of St Thomas'.[82] The Griffiths Report on Management drew on notions of her legendary exactitude to illustrate the extent of the need for good management in the NHS: 'If Florence Nightingale were carrying her lamp through the corridors of the NHS today, she would almost certainly be searching for the people in charge.' But no historical icon could stop the changes to training and work cultures as the implementation of *Project 2000* recommendations progressed.[83] Despite the discriminatory recruitment procedures, Graham Haynes had found the Nightingale School to be very different to other nursing schools he had worked in: 'it was wonderful to have this freedom and liberation of thought and deed and action in the Nightingale School, it really was quite revolutionary I think in its way of operating'. But by the late 1980s things became very difficult. The Director of Nursing Education left as she did not want to be involved in amalgamating the School with Guy's School of Nursing. Graham then became head of post-registration education working with Jane Easterbrook as acting director of nursing education. It was a time of flux and Graham recollects the frustration of writing and preparing new nursing curriculums for the nursing degree course as educators had been given only a three-month timeline.[84] In 1991, the Nightingale and Guy's College of Nursing and Midwifery was formed from the Nightingale School of Nursing and Thomas Guy and Lewisham School of Nursing. Consultation and collaboration with King's College London led to the first cohort of *Project 2000* nurses starting their Diploma in Higher Education in Nursing in October 1993.[85] Renamed the Nightingale and Guy's College of Health in 1993, it then joined with Normanby College of Health within King's College, its higher education base. The brochure produced to mark the merger contained historical details around the development of nursing in both institutions, and included images of the statues of Florence Nightingale and Thomas Guy.

Unsurprisingly there was strong resistance to the mergers of the three nursing schools. Institutional loyalties were as strong in nursing as in medicine. Guy's Nursing League had expressed concern when the creation of the Lewisham and North Southwark Health Authority omitted Guy's name from the title.[86] At St Thomas' nursing leaders were adamant that the Nightingale name should be used. Redundancies were inevitable and one interviewee reflected: 'I always think of it as being rather like a cull on the ice flow, some people were clubbed to death, others managed to swim and certainly there was a lot of blood on the ice at that time.'[87] In the initial period, the lack of provision of accommodation at King's College for nursing education staff meant that teaching took place in gyms, churches, and even a conservatory attached to a garden centre. Nursing educators invested in suitcases with wheels as that was the only practical way of transporting large quantities of teaching material across multiple sites during the day. Logistical problems also ensued, with incompatible computer systems and the academic summer shutdown at King's conflicting with the nurses' year-round education demands.

Reflecting on the long-term consequences of *Project 2000* and the relocation of nurse training to a university campus, Sue Norman, who had been Nurse Tutor at St Thomas' between 1987 and 1987, believed that nurse educators had more control over the student experience during the earlier period.[88] Natalie Tiddy, who had fought very hard to stop nursing and midwifery going to a university base, noted how the changes served to disconnect nurses and other staff from the hospital that was their workplace.

People training in university don't have the affiliation with the hospital they had when you trained within the hospital. That was your sort of centre. Now that isn't. Because they train at St Thomas', King's, Lewisham, wherever, they can have no affiliation to any one particular site or any one particular section because they've been all over, so that's their training. Their affiliation is to the university… But of course, they don't work for it. They're on an educational study. They're living on a grant or whatever it is, so they're not working for anybody, they don't have the responsibility to that organisation, and that's what I feel has gone wrong.[89]

But others perceived that the changes helped students become more patient-focused even though they had to complete more postgraduate learning.[90]

Making heritage visible

The history of the two institutions had interwoven through every aspect of everyday life in the hospitals and training schools since the nineteenth century. It is unsurprising then that during the 1980s, when mergers brought forth new fears about the loss of institutional identities, there were initiatives to preserve and promote the heritage more widely. At Guy's the Gordon Museum had been founded in the early twentieth century through an endowment from Mr Robert Gordon. Focused on pathology and housing specimens dating from the work of historical figures including Richard Bright, Thomas Addison, and Thomas Hodgkin, the Museum was an invaluable teaching resource for students and was part of institutional history. Tina Challacombe, Guy's alumnus, reflected on the relationship between history and institutional name.

Well, I suppose when we came to Guy's Hospital, it was very much the traditions that had gone before that were brought to your attention, as students, and the famous physicians and surgeons that had worked here, all the names of the wards, the names of the lecture theatres and the Gordon Museum with all the wonderful specimens, constantly reminded you of the past name and history and heritage and there was a real worry, probably unfounded, that that might get lost a bit in the changes of the name. I mean, I know it's only a name and that Guy's Hospital stands forever, but I think there was a perception among one's colleagues, at that time, that it was going to be lost and enveloped in another name and I'm proud to be part of Guy's Hospital, if you read a lot of books, history books, literature books and they talk about hospitals and medicine … we travel the world to different conferences, nearly everybody we meet has heard of Guy's Hospital, so we are very proud of that heritage that we represent.[91]

In 1982 St Thomas' founded the Florence Nightingale Museum Trust with the launch of a public appeal to raise the initial £500k to build, equip, and endow the Museum and Resources Centre.[92] The aim was the creation of a museum at St Thomas', where the Nightingale Training School held a collection of 'Nightingalia'. The collection had grown under the guardianship of Dame Alicia Lloyd-Still during her time as Matron of St Thomas' Hospital between 1913 and 1937.[93] The plans for a dedicated museum were timely, as a 'heritage boom' was underway. An unprecedented number of heritage institutions opened during the Thatcher years, from visitor centres and museums to living history sites where the past was re-created. The boom is especially associated with industrial heritage – as manufacturing sites closed, their workers fought to preserve their past; however, many independent museums also formed links to professions beyond manufacturing.[94] Against this backdrop, the Nightingale Museum was leased land from the hospital on the site of the original nursing school for a 'peppercorn rent'. Patricia Mowbray,

Art Historian, remembers John Wyn Owen asking her if it would be viable to found a St Thomas' Museum. She recalls saying, 'No, but you could have a Florence Nightingale Museum tomorrow.'[95] Patricia and John Wyn Owen were joined by Mary Laurence, the chief nurse, and Natalie Tiddy. A major fundraising initiative was launched with approaches to businesses, alumni and even army regiments who had received honours from the Crimean War: 'money flowed in, on a wing and a prayer, I was always optimistic and never brooded if something went wrong,' reflected Patricia, who was a member of the Events Committee.[96] The scale of the fundraising illustrates St Thomas' deep networks across the great and the good. One of the first events was a sold-out concert by the Gabriele String Quartet, held in Goldsmiths' Hall, which raised over £7,000.[97] Natalie recalls that not all staff welcomed the establishment of the museum – which created anguish amongst medical staff over the loss of their car park, whilst the museum's advocates felt this location was significant. Although unfamiliar to Florence, it would have been in view of her apartments. Natalie explains the museum grew from an impulse to preserve and display Nightingale's heritage: 'to have something like Florence Nightingale as part of our direct heritage and not to actually share that when we found all this stuff up in the attic just seemed criminal. Absolutely criminal'.[98] As the Royal College of Nurses and unions campaigned for better pay and recognition, the historic and contemporary importance of their role in society could be seen by the public when the museum opened in 1989. A life-size recreation of a ward at Scutari was the centrepiece, and fundraising was continuing to support grant awards to nurses wishing to undertake postgraduate studies.

> Now it's going ahead in leaps and bounds. It's wonderful. Since it was first opened it's now been renovated and upgraded, and we've managed to raise over £1 million to get the upgrading done. So, it goes to show there is still an interest in Florence Nightingale. And while it remains

in the curriculum for primary school children it will exist.
If that goes, the Museum won't be sustained because it's
completely self-funding.[99]

Patients, clinicians, and communications

Paternalistic cultures had shaped medicine and patient care since the
professionalisation of medicine in the nineteenth century. By the 1980s
a new emphasis on patient autonomy had emerged from feminist
debates. These expressed wide concern about the entanglements
between biomedicine and male dominance, which prevented patients
from making decisions about their own healthcare. The burgeoning
of new therapies and technologies in the postwar period had created
a social expectation that medicine could cure every condition under
the sun and led to a rising demand for healthcare. Cyril Chantler
noted that when he qualified in the 1960s, the question asked by
patients was 'what can be done?'; doctors operated as 'independent
advisers concerned with diseases'.[100] Rationing of new technologies
such as kidney dialysis because of limited resources was undertaken
by consultant doctors as described in Chapter 3. The 1980s was a
critical time of change as patients and their advocates became more
vocal about the need for clinicians to embrace the patient as a person
and move away from a paternalistic, disease-focused approach.

Better care for dying patients was pioneered by Dame Cicely
Saunders through the setting up of St Christopher's Hospice in the
late 1960s but the growth of hospices had been limited by the financial
constraints of the late 1970s.[101] Thelma Bates joined St Thomas'
as consultant in radiotherapy in 1968, and in 1978 the department
had moved to a purpose-designed space in the newly built North
Wing. Thelma was motivated by 'the quality of care' delivered by
the hospice movement to consider how to improve the care given to
end-of-life patients within St Thomas'. 'No one was happy with the

existing standard of terminal care at St Thomas',' she concluded after early discussions with consultants and nurses. The Special Trustees agreed to fund the establishment of a multidisciplinary consultative team which included the hospital chaplain. The team worked with consultants and patients across the hospital and in the community with district nurses and GPs, and this challenged some of the norms of the time where consultants and GPs believed it was unnecessary to have other clinicians involved in the care of their patients. 'It was the first of its kind in the UK. It was copied internationally and became the first academic department of Palliative Medicine in the UK in 1991,' noted Thelma.[102]

The HIV/AIDS crisis of the 1980s was an important moment in the longer history of patient activism as the work of self-help groups brought about important changes in access to drugs and the design and management of clinical trials.[103] The medical focus on disease management and the lack of engagement with holistic patient care and appreciation of the social changes around sexuality is starkly illustrated in the treatment of Terrence (Terry) Higgins. Terry was a computer programmer in his 30s and after collapsing on the dancefloor during a night out was taken to St Thomas' by ambulance in 1982. Rupert Whitaker, his partner, visited him but struggled to get any information from medical staff.

> Well I remember going in to visit Terry and he was in an isolation unit at the time and I was only allowed to look at him through a window, nobody was allowed in, there was complete barrier nursing, and I was not really allowed to know what was going on, I don't think the staff really knew what was going on, but Terry had been just sort of brought in on an emergency and quickly isolated because there was a suspicion, as I understand it, that there was some risk of infection.

After the initial quarantine period, Terry was occasionally discharged but his health gradually worsened, and he died at St Thomas' on 4 July 1982. Rupert was only 19 years old at the time and could not get information about the cause of Terry's death.

> Terry had no immediate family, and his friends and I were the ones who were most in touch, well we were the only ones who were in touch, and even after he died nobody would tell me what he'd died of, although we knew, and I had asked his consultant physician at the time, in writing, as we were setting up the Terrence Higgins Trust, if he could confirm in writing what Terry died of. But the consultant physician didn't recognise my relationship to Terry at all, even though his body had been released to me. I had to pay for the funeral out of my student grant, and I had to organise the funeral, and it was this complete disconnect between the body and the person of Terry and who he was and what his friends meant to him and what he meant to us.

A year or so later, Rupert ran into some of the clinicians who had treated Terry:

> First of all they were very surprised that I was still alive because I had been sick myself. Then I said, you know, we still want absolute confirmation about what Terry had when he died and what he died of in particular. And they said, 'well we've written up the autopsy and we're publishing it in either the *Lancet* or the *BMJ* and you can read what he died of in there'. [the physicians] were to my mind too busy playing doctor to be good physicians, and it's been a lifelong experience for me about physicians who just don't know how to relate and how to look at the reality of illness and their patients' lives.[104]

The distressing aspects of Terry's care contributed to Rupert's decision to establish the Terrence Higgins Trust, alongside Martyn Butler. The Trust was created with 'the intention of preventing others from having to suffer as Terry had'. It grew to support research, direct-support, education and awareness of AIDS and HIV – described in the early 1980s as Gay-Related Immune Deficiency.[105]

David Barlow specialised in genitourinary medicine (GUM) and remembers those early days.

> Looking back at the level of ignorance that we knew about managing HIV and its complications…there were of course no antiretroviral drugs, we couldn't grow the virus in those days. We knew there was a thing called the gay compromise syndrome, because it was largely gay men it seemed who'd got it…in those days medically speaking people didn't understand what was going on at all.

After a visit to San Francisco General Hospital in 1985, David established the first dedicated outpatient unit for HIV at St Thomas'.

> We had a chest physician, we had a skin physician, we had an eye doctor, we had a neurologist. All the people would come to our clinic so that the HIV positive patients, who were largely gay men or injecting drug users, largely from abroad or African folk, had all those services laid on this floor. So instead of saying you need to go and see a skin doctor and have to go off somewhere else in the hospital… it was a really important…it was never given as much credit. I think ten years later people are realising that in fact you should deliver the service to the patient rather than the patient having to go and find the service. So that was actually quite an important innovation, which was at St Thomas'.

During this period David was the administrative head of the GUM department and describes the complexities of the role as clinical management was adopted.

> I suddenly found I'd got a finance director and I'd got a business manager…looking after me and maybe a couple of others. Suddenly I had somebody else to write the business plan. Otherwise, I was doing research, I was publishing a lot of stuff, I was lecturing, I was involved with the medical students. I was a busy person in those days. But doing the business plan and working out how you were going to spend the money of the department was part of what one did.

There was a lot of additional funding for HIV and AIDS, and David found himself in 'a very strong negotiating position' as everyone wanted his money, but clinical management structures enabled him to ringfence it for research activities.

> In purely practical terms it was a very exciting time to be managing a department, because there was a lot of HIV and AIDS money. There was a huge, largely gay man driven pressure to make sure that HIV, AIDS was properly funded. We had the largest number of heterosexual HIV patients in the country. I didn't have a formal training, and I've never been an academic, but I've done a lot of research. I'm particularly interested in epidemiology and the transmission of disease, and I took a particular interest in how HIV was transmitted heterosexually and whether it was a problem in this country.[106]

Meanwhile, Rupert Whitaker's distressing experience of Terry Higgins' care led him to gain expertise in psychology, neurology, and immunology and become a consultant in psychiatry and medical science. He continues to advocate for the biopsychosocial model of medicine, which addresses all the domains of the body, mind, and the person in context.

> You do tend to get a consensus among clinicians because they know the way they've done it, and they know the way they'd like to do it. It may or may not be and usually isn't particularly relevant to what needs to be done from the patient's perspective. And that is the problem of culture also, of professional culture, so the problem is that with this consensus amongst clinicians and the way things are... this is the way we do things, and this is the way it should be done, you need to break that, you need to break that framework and start it from scratch.[107]

Like Rupert, one mother whose child was treated for kidney failure at Guy's – Helen Lewis – had a similarly life-changing experience of hospital care. This led Helen to eventually gain a PhD in sociology through studying patient and carer experiences of children receiving renal care in hospital. In 1980 her child had been taken seriously ill and was transferred to the children's kidney unit at Guy's after spending several weeks at Great Ormond Street Children's Hospital. Haemodialysis was the initial treatment but was soon changed to Continuous Peritoneal Dialysis (CPD) at home, so that her child could attend school with her peer group, otherwise support for parents was minimal.

> In those early days, you could sleep overnight in the hospital, but you slept in the children's dining room...you had to make up your own bed and you had to get your own sheets... And there was no food or anything for parents. The food was there for the children. So, you were going out and buying snacks in Borough High Street...you were subsisting really. So, I slept on the hospital ward Monday to

Friday nights and my husband came up at weekends. We had a son. My mother came down from Yorkshire to look after him. She was widowed by then, and she was able to stay. So, we managed that stage.

The decision was then taken to proceed with a kidney transplant with the kidney donated by the mother, which lasted until the child was 11. A second transplant failed, and a third transplant lasted until her daughter reached her mid-twenties, when she went on to CPD again until her death in 1999. During the early years there was no acknowledgement of the psychological and emotional impact of chronic disease on children and carers: 'the biggest thing you take away really is the fear. And you have to live with that fear, and the child has to live with the fear'. Her reminiscences of the experience of being in the clinic with other parents waiting for test results that could often take a whole day to arrive speak strongly to the dissonance in doctor-patient relationships. As an articulate, highly-educated woman she was able to communicate with doctors in a way that many distressed parents could not and left them vulnerable to misunderstanding their child's care regimes.

So, it was about then developing a working relationship with the medical staff. Because there was a culture in the waiting room, which you quickly see, of parents not understanding what's going on and not feeling able to challenge what's going on, or even able to phrase the right question to find out what's going on. Because if you think it's at a time, the 1980s, when all sorts of social changes were taking place. So, the generation older than us, who had not had the NHS there all their lives, had an attitude of gratitude to their doctor and, an attitude of – I don't want to bother the doctor, we're very grateful for his care. And I think society changed and I suppose I was lucky to have had an education which was as good as a medical education, so I didn't actually feel intimidated by doctors. And I think a lot of mothers did. There were people who didn't know how to ask.

Helen's powerful awareness of the need for change led to her undertaking research into patients' and carers' experiences of children's renal disease, and for those who survived their experience of transition into adulthood.

> I did a survey, sending a thousand questionnaires to patients in transition to adulthood in 14 hospitals in the UK. I funded it myself. Afterwards, I did 40 interviews with patients and then 20 with parents. But I knew what questions I wanted to ask, and I knew what questions medicine needed to address. And that came from the Guy's experience and the whole attitude that life returns to normal after transplantation.[108]

Becoming Trusts

Margaret Thatcher initially asked the think-tank, the Centre for Policy Studies, headed by David Willetts, to review the NHS in 1987. This was followed in January 1988 by her making an unexpected public announcement on the BBC Panorama programme that there would be wider NHS review carried out behind closed doors with no input from clinicians. The outcome was the White Paper, *Working for Patients (WfP)*. Guy's and St Thomas' clinicians with strong political networks were too savvy to desist from influencing decisions from afar. David Willetts, for example, visited Guy's during the period, and Ian McColl, Professor of Surgery, showed him the commemorative plaque which recorded the last Board of Governors' meeting at Guy's in 1974. It was a stark reminder that teaching hospitals lost their boards of governors under the Conservatives in 1974, not Labour in 1948.[109] *WfP*, which was published in January 1989, introduced a quasi-market into the NHS by separating the bodies who provided care from those who purchased it. Funding allocation was to be based on population, with adjustments for the age and morbidity, as opposed to historic allocation with the money following the patient. In August 1989, Kenneth Clarke was appointed Secretary of State for Health and Social Care. Clarke, who had been involved in the 1974 reorganisation, was critical of consensus management and strongly advocated devolved decision-making.

The most significant aspect of the reforms for Guy's and St Thomas' was the option for acute hospitals to apply for self-governing status through becoming trusts. Trusts would be funded directly from government with accountability given to the Board of Trustees. The initiative was part of a wider government agenda focused on improving efficiency through devolved accountability. Karen Caines was a civil servant in Margaret Thatcher's Efficiency Unit in the 1980s and worked on the development of the *Next Steps Report* on the wider civil service. This 1988 paper has been regarded as a 'quiet revolution' in service management, which advocated the division of the civil service, extracting those with policy and ministerial responsibilities from the majority of civil servants who would in turn be divided into semi-autonomous agencies with chief executives managing targets.[110] Karen then became involved in the establishment of NHS Trusts, and recollects the sense of independence that trust status was anticipated to provide.

> My reading is, the London teaching hospitals, Guy's, Thomas', Bart's, had had exactly those kind of freedoms under the Board of Governors, not that long before…So, there was a sense in which, for a lot of the staff at Guy's, certainly a lot of the clinicians, this did not come as some fancy new management theory, this was, well this is the natural way of the world, now we're getting back where we should be, and we never really understood all these District Health Authorities and stuff but now we're Guy's.[111]

As part of the implementation of *WfP*, the South East Thames RHA had set up a project group on self-governing hospitals with the aim of screening initial candidates, supporting the preparation of business plans, undertaking local consultation, and giving detailed advice to the Secretary of State for Health. The intention was that applications for self-governing status would be made immediately following the enactment of the legislation with trusts becoming established in April 1991. The Department of Health had provided 'substantial' financial resources to support these preparations, including £32 million on 5 June 1989 of which £1.9 million was allocated to the RHA.

At Guy's, the management team pressed ahead with preparations despite strong resistance from some consultants that Trust status would be instrumental in enabling privatisation of the NHS: the idea of Trusts was 'utterly opposed' by some members of the Lewisham and North Southwark Health Authority and 'half the medical body... it was a terrible, miserable time,' remembered Elaine Murphy who was then Acting District General Manager.[112] Professor Harry Keen, Director of the Unit for Metabolic Medicine and Director of Clinical Services/Medicine for Guy's Hospital was so opposed to the idea on the basis that it would fuel the privatisation agenda, that in December 1989 he applied for judicial review on the grounds that it was unlawful to expend the resources, financial and other, that were being spent on the preparations before the Bill became law.

> Within Guy's Hospital there is considerable controversy as to the desirability of Guy's Hospital making this change in its status. A ballot of Guy's Hospital's consultants was held on the question and of 213 consultants eligible to vote, 107 returned the ballot papers, 30 supported the Guy's Hospital's decision to 'express an interest', 71 opposed it and six expressed no view either way. Considerable scepticism was expressed by the hospitals' medical and dental committee on 9 May 1989.[113]

Keen's application for judicial review was dismissed on 21 February 1990, but the reforms were politically polarised and divided opinions across Guy's: 'as fervent as Ian McColl was about the Conservative party, Harry [Keen] was as fervent for the Labour Party, and felt that these reforms were the first major step to privatisation of the NHS and should be opposed'.[114] Nevertheless, plans proceeded and various interviewees related that the consultant body had been won over by the promise of additional funding for the Phase 3 building of Philip Harris House, which began in July 1990.

Guy's joined with Lewisham Hospital in the run-up to Trust application which brought significant strengths in terms of an increased patient population. Professor Maurice Lessof, clinical immunologist and deputy Chairman of Guy's and Lewisham Trust (1991-1993), described moving his team to Lewisham as a means of establishing good relationships.

> So that there was a professorial team at Lewisham working for them... this wasn't a takeover of the teaching by the teaching hospital. It was a partnership. And six months later, Ian McColl, later Lord McColl, brought the surgical team down, did the same thing.[115]

Guy's innovative adoption of clinical directorate management chimed with political ideologies and Guy's and Lewisham became the 'flagship' NHS Trust when the first wave of hospitals to be granted trust status was announced in December 1990.[116] Its position as the Government's 'flagship' was strengthened by the appointment of Peter Griffiths as Chief Executive. Peter had joined the NHS Administrator Training Scheme after leaving school. He had worked his way through administration/management roles becoming District Administrator, and then District General Manager of Lewisham and North Southwark Health Authority in the 1980s. At that point he became involved with Guy's and aware of how depressed the clinicians were at the quality of management of the hospital. He was part of the group led by Cyril Chantler that had visited Johns Hopkins in the US during 1984 to learn about their models of clinical directorates. In 1988/89 Peter was invited to undertake a secondment at the Department of Health to establish NHS Trusts in England and was initially responsible for the Trusts programme before becoming Deputy Chief Executive of the Management Executive at the Department of Health, with oversight for health services across England.

> My task, when I arrived in the Management Executive, in the first instance, was to take the idea of self-governing hospitals and help create what that would mean in detail, really, and create a programme, national programme, for the establishment of what were to become the first wave of NHS Trusts.

The chair of the new Trust was Philip Harris, now Lord Harris, former chief executive of the carpet company, Harris Queensway, deputy treasurer of the Conservative Party and a major investor in Guy's genes and cancer units. He remembered the constant media attention.

> We were in the newspapers I think everywhere, the flagship, because Guy's was determined to do that, it was controversial and got listed about that in all sorts of places. But we were planning to be the first NHS Trust and a certain amount of this went on behind closed doors.[117]

Karen Caines, who moved from the civil service to take up the post of General Manager at Guy's in 1991, recalls that 'in some people's eyes, it wasn't Guy's as a hospital, like Tommy's, like Bart's, like whatever...it was kind of emblematic of a Thatcherite set of reforms'.[118] Trust status fed into deeply-embedded ambitions about quality, she noted.

> So, there was a lot of thinking going on everywhere, about quality, and I think that played to Guy's own sense of feeling itself to be a quality institution and wanting to be. With all these reforms, you know, reforms are great when you're doing it to somebody, and it's not so great when it's being done to you. But a lot of this, I think, did genuinely feel to people in Guy's, this is getting rid of the nameless bureaucracy above us, which we never understood anyway, and now we can do it…but the Trust provided a stimulus.[119]

Headhunted and appointed as the Trust's new Director of Nursing, Wilma MacPherson had previously been working across Grampian, which provided services across the North East of Scotland including Orkney and Shetland. On arrival she found 'things that were excellent and other things that surprised me because they were not quite so good'. From an outsider's perspective, the need for Trusts in London was obvious: 'You'd so many different places competing for the same little pot and the actual population had gone down quite dramatically.'[120]

But very rapidly the new Trust's status changed as a budgetary 'blackhole' caused the management team to take swift and effective action to stem financial losses through redundancies and cutbacks. Every clinical service was to be evaluated in terms of its relevance to local health needs and efficiency. The initial announcement of up to 600 redundancies amounting to almost 10 per cent of the workforce was made by Peter Griffiths in May 1991: the Trust 'has to sort itself out this year', he stated. It wanted to clear its debts of £6.8 million and invest a further £6 million in its 'most important' staff and services.[121] In retrospect the communication of Trust's plans was 'absolutely agonising, and very badly handled PR'.[122] The underlying cause for the cuts was the need for the hospital to adjust to the dynamics of the internal market and the pressure of competition. But those who had opposed the hospital's move to Trust status viewed the cuts as a direct consequence: the Trust was being run like a 'banana republic. Consultants were told that Trust status would mean greater prosperity and that money would be coming in. We are aghast as the proposed redundancies,' said Harry Keen.[123] The announcement coincided with the May 1991 County council elections in which the Conservatives lost hundreds of seats. Conservative evaluation showed that a large percentage of respondents said that they had voted against the Conservatives because of the redundancies at the Trust. Chief Executive Peter Griffiths was called to account.

> I was informally summoned to talk to a number of Conservative backbenchers and other people to check out whether I was a raging communist because I had inflicted such personal damage on the Government of the day.

The media spotlight was intense. Peter was followed by reporters and remembers 'the intense personal animosity [in media reports] and intense personal influence on my family and so on, which was extremely unpleasant and quite prolonged'.[124] Wilma MacPherson, Director of Nursing, recollected that, 'everybody was watching Guy's and Lewisham, like hawks. We had *The Sun* photographers hiding in bushes to take photos of people's cars…even David Brindle [journalist] put a bit about me in *The Guardian*, because I had been fairly vocal at the [Royal College of Nursing] about the risks of trusts, so he was playing it back to me'.[125]

Phil Harris remained undaunted by the challenges and remembered how rapidly the team was able to turn things around.

> I went through the complete budget, and we had a £3 million overspend, and we looked at how we could do it.

It meant 600 people had to go and of course, they all said it was doctors and nurses; it wasn't. We had marches and social protests, and we all went through it, we didn't give in, I wouldn't give in because it was the right thing to do by the way, it wasn't the wrong thing. We did miss them [the staff] when they went, miss paying them. We did balance the books. The first year was about £6 million, the second year we had £20 million surplus and we've spent money on buildings as well...so we went from doing everything wrong for 18 months to everything right. I think the two things I remember, apart from having a fantastic time, was the unions actually agreed that it was better, which was unbelievable, when they left us alone. Everyone was on side at the end, and getting Lewisham and Guy's to work together was very important as well.[126]

The new culture of NHS Trusts led to income generation activities being extended. Revenue generation had been adopted in the 1980s as a means of producing additional income to supplement the reduction in budgets. Lee Soden worked at Guy's as District Catering Manager in the late 1970s and early 1980s. He left in 1985 to work in the private sector for Gardner Merchant, one of the external contractors working to secure NHS catering contracts, returning in 1989 as Director of Commercial Services: 'I brought a different commercial acumen to what I was doing at Guy's and even to this day I still believe that all those years on, having left the health service and went out into the commercial world and brought that expertise back is the best thing I ever did.' His work was split across catering and commercial services with the aim of generating income for the hospital: 'it was a way of saying, well if you can't get the money because the Government want to cut down, we'll go and get the money by selling our services to others and then bringing the money back in'.[127] In December 1992 the first McDonald's burger restaurant opened on the Guy's site and despite initial criticism that McDonald's did not offer healthy food, it was a highly successful venture: 'This is in keeping with our Trust Charter commitment to improve conditions for staff,' noted Chairman Philip Harris.[128] The Robens Suite at the top of Guy's Tower with its unsurpassable views of St Paul's was developed into a highly successful hospitality suite, and the provision of support across medical, non-medical, and catering areas to other countries including Saudi Arabia and Kazakhstan, proved successful in generating income.

In February 1992, Karen Caines wrote a position paper on Guy's management philosophy for discussion with the Executive team. The key proposition was that Guy's was 'too large, complex, diverse and professional an organisation to be run prescriptively from any central point, whether clinical or managerial'.

> In essence what makes Guy's great is the quality of a single moment of professional judgement, repeated over and over again by large numbers of people in different professions. That moment of judgement may be informed by knowledge and experience, but it is always individual and always unique. It cannot be determined centrally. To be successful, we have to foster individualism, decisiveness, entrepreneurialism.

The paper suggested a slimline corporate framework that would give strategic direction and a 'very few' robust managerial rules of the game that would define the ends rather than the means.[129] As the Trust got to grips with the restructuring of the Clinical Directorates with the specific aim of liberating them to fulfil their potential, service innovations were rapidly set-up to benefit patients.

> Simple little things like ante-natal clinics, renting a space in Lewisham Shopping Centre, so that pregnant women, many of whom will have another child, didn't have to

haul up on the train to London Bridge or some long bus ride...it makes a huge difference to people's expectations and experiences of hospitals. And putting on ante-natal clinics early in the morning, and in late afternoon, and we were wanting to move into evening for people who were working...the clinicians were great, they wanted it.[130]

The positivity of the period even extended to patients' food choices as Guy's collaborated with Claudia Roden, specialist in Middle Eastern and Italian cooking, and Caroline Waldegrave, principal of Leith's School of Food and Wine, and wife to William Waldegrave, Secretary of State for Health, to develop new menus for patients. Food writers including Josceline Dimbleby were invited to contribute recipes to create a 14-day menu of 28 different meals. Head chef Ettore Eligio, who had joined Guy's from Claridge's so that he could spend more time with his children, reflected that the new menu made him feel like cooking again. Even though entirely fresh products were used, Gary McKenna, general manager of catering services, noted that the costs were within the daily patient food allowance of £1.79.[131] And the topping out ceremony for the building of Philip Harris House, carried out on 24 July 1991, reassured staff that despite the difficulties, the future of Guy's and Lewisham NHS Trust was rosy.

Whereas Guy's had enjoyed the benefits of being the Government's flagship Trust, St Thomas' experience of applying for Trust status was very different. The financial pressures of the 1980s had brought the hospital to the brink and in February 1990 a majority of the consultant staff opposed the move to opt-out.[132] In November 1990 the hospital's application to become a Trust was refused on the grounds that it was not financially robust: 'the move will undoubtedly throw another question mark over whether St Thomas' should be closed,' noted the *Times* correspondent in November 1990.[133] Nevertheless, Neil Hooper, finance director at St Thomas', affirmed that it had made 'incredible progress' as through a combination of cost improvement programmes, income generation schemes, and rationalisation of manpower, it had reduced the monthly overspend of £400,000 in January 1990 to a monthly underspend of between £100,000 to £200,000.[134] The appointment of Sir Robert Reid as chairman in that year was instrumental in steering St Thomas' through the turbulent waters of this period. Sir Robert had forged his career in the railway industry, becoming chairman of British Rail in 1983 and successfully delivering efficiencies in the context of its anticipated privatisation. In 1990 he was offered the chairman role at St Thomas' by Peter Griffiths who at that time worked at the NHS Management Executive.

> I was concerned that I knew very little about how hospitals were run, let alone a traditional institution such as St Thomas'. Within months of joining, I was faced with the task of finding a new Chief Executive and building a strong management team. We had to alter the generally held opinion that St Thomas' was not worth helping.[135]

The new appointee to St Thomas' was Tim Matthews who had built his career in health management through junior appointments in the Department of Health and Social Security where he worked on NHS reforms and then general manager appointments in London and Kent.[136] On 1 June 1991 he was appointed as general manager to West Lambeth Health Authority and as the chief executive designate for St Thomas' with a remit of completing the process of separating out the hospitals from the health authority prior to setting up St Thomas' as a Trust in its own right.

> At that time there was no explicit prospect of a merger…so the remit was to stabilise St Thomas' financially, because it had come through quite a rocky financial period to ensure that we achieved Trust status as an independent hospital and grow it and develop it effectively.

Under the previous leadership of Stephen Jenkins, St Thomas' had undergone a financial restructuring with the creation of seven directorates each headed by a member of the new Executive Management Team. Tim inherited 'a good team' and in September 1991 was able to reassure readers of the West Lambeth Authority's staff magazine *Circle* that, 'our financial position is strong, and many tough decisions have already been taken and their consequences faced'.[137] He also provided reassurances that the re-application to become a Trust would not affect patient care nor have adverse impact on staff pay or conditions. The financial pressures of the early 1990s were viewed by many as a new and contemporary problem. But Wyndham Lloyd-Davies, surgeon at St Thomas', used his 1992 Presidential Address to the British Association of Urological Surgeons to contextualise current pressures in the longer history of St Thomas'. He was proud of being the 'eighth in line father to son in medicine' and reviewed the financial crises suffered by St Thomas' since the fourteenth and fifteenth centuries: 'we may all take heart from the fact that our present problems have been around for a very long time'. He reviewed how urology and lithotripsy services had been managed since the late 1980s and the change in financial control from functional budgeting – costs split across nursing, medical and administration aspects – to clinical budgeting and resource management. Since 1989, the budgets for urology and lithotripsy services had been separated, enabling comparisons between services and across periods. The concept of clinical directors controlling their departmental budgets was 'the undoubted way forward in modern hospital management' and the next stage would be 'to break down all costs and itemise services as is being done so successfully in the Royal Liverpool University Trust Department of Urology'. He was in no doubt that rationalising budgets to finance the new and expensive treatments was a 'painful and difficult task' but one that could not be shirked by either governments or hospitals. Indeed, it was the heritage of St Thomas' that would enable it to meet the challenges.[138]

During this early period as newly-formed Trusts, Guy's and Lewisham, and St Thomas' focused on addressing the challenges of Trust status and planning for the future. There was no indication that future plans would implode because of the wider reconfiguration of London health services.

Conclusion

By the end of the 1980s, every branch of Guy's and St Thomas' – medical, dental, and nursing schools and the hospitals – had been forced to engage with major changes to their structures and processes. The medical schools' merger was initially only implemented for the administration of the schools, and it was several years before the separate teaching programmes were reconfigured. Given the unhappiness caused by the merger of students' sports activities, it is no surprise that there was no rush to implement the merger across the schools. Merging the nursing schools proved to be more contentious than the merger of the medical schools. This was largely because the merger was implemented swiftly and the wider changes across the wider landscape of nurse training with *Project 2000*, which sought to change the basis of nurse training into higher education institutions, were hugely unsettling. On paper, the mergers appeared to have brought the institutions closer together. But the hospitals had followed very different trajectories during the 1980s, particularly regarding the challenges of managing cuts and cash limits and the process of becoming Trusts. The 1990s were to bring the biggest challenge yet with the proposed merger of Guy's and St Thomas' Trusts as part of the wider changes across London.

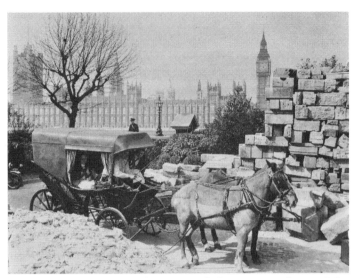

1. St Thomas' Hospital: return of Florence Nightingale's carriage to the hospital, 1942, image © London Metropolitan Archives (City of London).

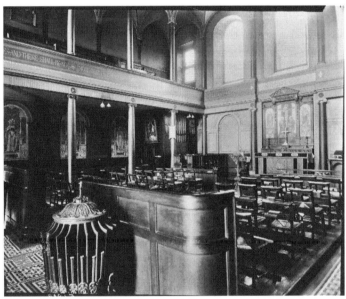

2. Guy's Hospital: chapel, interior, 1968, image © London Metropolitan Archives (City of London).

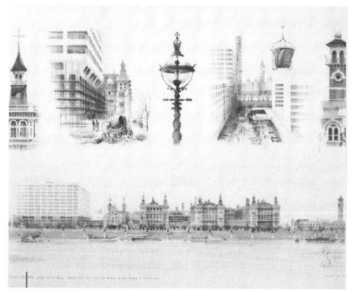

3. St Thomas' Hospital Under Construction, 1975, lithograph, S2000.87 © David Gentleman.

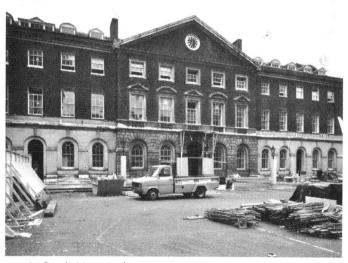

4. Guy's Hospital: exterior, 1980, image © London Metropolitan Archives (City of London). (also used on back book cover)

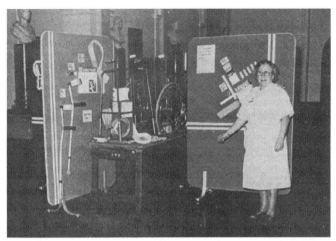

5. The first 'What It Costs' exhibition on Physiotherapy in Central Hall, St Thomas' Hospital showing Miss Maureen Dillon, Superintendent Physiotherapist who initiated the idea. Image taken from *Circle: The Magazine for the St Thomas' Health District (Teaching)*, 1980.

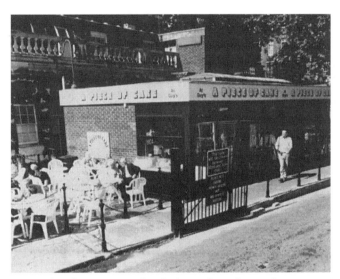

6. A Piece of Cake, a specialist baker of quality cakes, pastries and breads, was an early income generation initiative at Guy's Hospital. Image taken from The Guy's Hospital Nurses' Ball Programme, 12 July 1991.

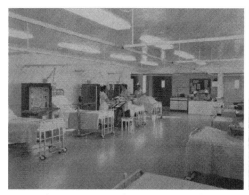

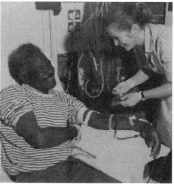

7. The new Renal Unit at Lambeth Hospital opened in August 1969 and ran initially as 5-day unit including night dialysis © Marianne Vennegoor.

8. Renal nursing education session underway at the Renal Unit, Lambeth Hospital c.1970s © Marianne Vennegoor.

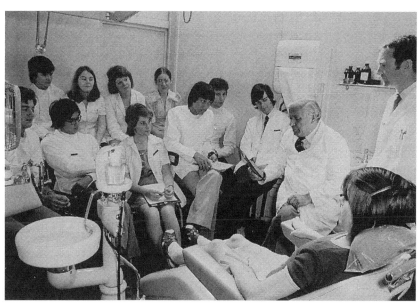

9. Jack Tulley, Professor of Orthodontics and Dean 1980-1985, teaching dental students at Guy's c. late 1970s/early 1980s © Gordon Museum, King's College London.

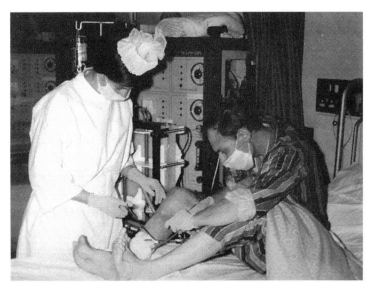

10. Brian Marchant, dialysis patient at St Thomas', c.1970
© Brian Marchant. (also used on front book cover)

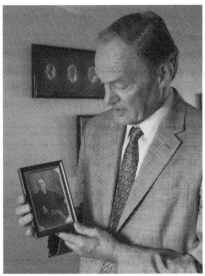

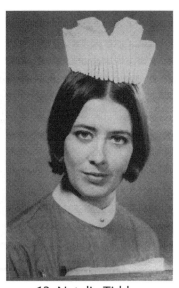

11. Medicine across the generations: Richard Hughes, Emeritus Professor of Neurology, Guy's, holding a portrait of Robert Hughes his great grandfather who was also a Guy's alumnus © Julian Simpson.

12. Natalie Tiddy, Nightingale Nurse c.1960s © Natalie Tiddy.

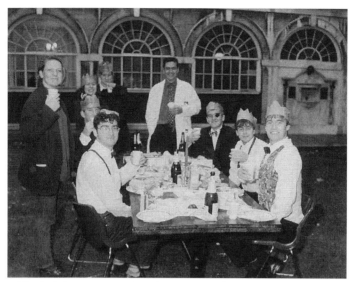

13. Celebrations in Guy's courtyard c.1980s © Gordon Museum, King's College London.

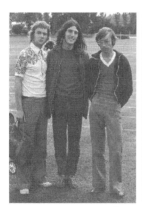

14. 30 years of service: Mike Messer (right) and colleagues at the St Thomas' Medical School, Annual Sports Day c.1970s © Mike Messer

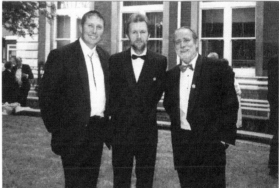

15. Mike Messer (right) and colleagues at a dinner to mark the end of teaching in Block Nine, St Thomas' c.2000s © Mike Messer.

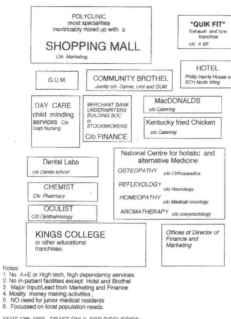

MODEL FOR A NON CLINICAL SECOND SITE

A conceptually coherent, ideologically indefensible,
community orientated money making facility

POLYCLINIC
most specialities
inextricably mixed up with a

SHOPPING MALL
C/o Marketing

"QUIK FIT"
Exhaust and tyre
franchise
c/o A &E

G.U.M.

COMMUNITY BROTHEL
Jointly c/o Gynae, Urol and GUM

HOTEL
Philip Harris House or
STH North Wing

DAY CARE
child minding
services C/o
Dept Nursing

MERCHANT BANK
UNDERWRITERS
BUILDING SOC
or
STOCKBROKERS
C/o FINANCE

MacDONALDS
c/o Catering

Kentucky fried Chicken
c/o Catering

Dental Labs
c/o Dental school

CHEMIST
C/o Pharmacy

OCULIST
C/o Ophthalmology

National Centre for holistic and
alternative Medicine

OSTEOPATHY c/o Orthopaedics

REFLEXOLOGY c/o Neurology

HOMEOPATHY c/o Medical oncology

AROMATHERAPY c/o coloproctology

KINGS COLLEGE
or other educational
franchisee.

Offices of Director of
Finance and
Marketing

Notes:
1. No A+E or High tech, high dependency services.
2. No in-patient facilities except Hotel and Brothel
3. Major Input/Lead from Marketing and Finance
4. Mostly money making activities ,
5. NO need for junior medical residents
6. Focussed on local population needs.

SEPT 13th 1993 DRAFT ONLY, FOR DISCUSSION ....

16. Spoof site plan created during the merger of Guy's and St Thomas' NHS Trusts, c.1990s.

17. Campaign poster for Save Guy's and St Thomas' Hospitals c.1990s © Marianne Vennegoor.

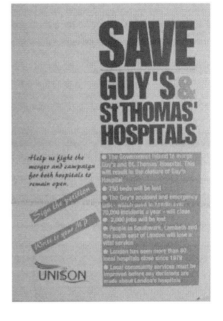

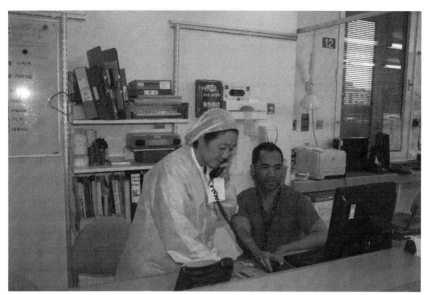

18. Christopher Bramaje and Cecilia Saquing at work, Guy's and St Thomas' NHS Foundation Trust, 2014 © Julian Simpson.

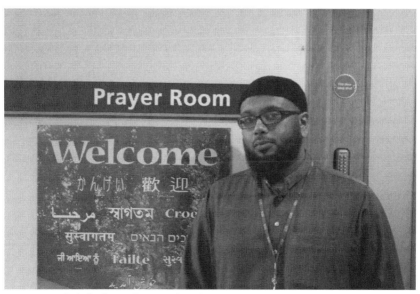

19. Abdul Chowdhury, chaplain, Guy's and St Thomas' NHS Foundation Trust, 2013 © Julian Simpson.

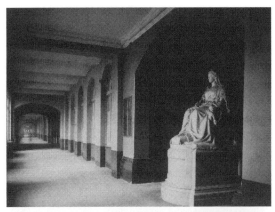

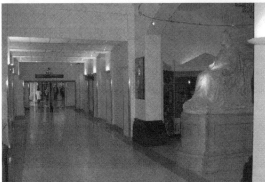

20. South Wing Corridor, St Thomas' Hospital c.1900 and 2007
© Mike Messer

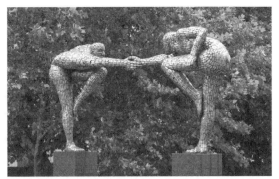

21. Commissioned for the millennium this piece symbolises the
relationships of trust and help that exist between patient and healer,
and the joining together of Guy's and St Thomas' hospitals. Cross
the Divide, 2000 © Rick Kirby. (also used on back book cover)

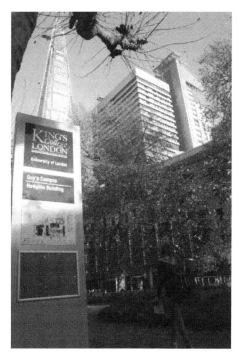

22. Guy's Campus, King's
College London,
2013 © Julian Simpson.

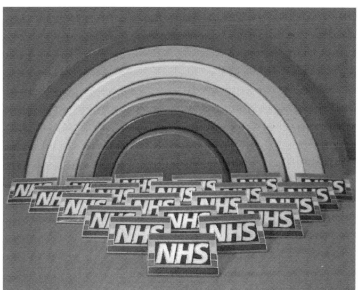

23. Rainbow badge initiated by Dr Michael Farquhar, consultant,
Evelina London, 2019 © Michael Farquhar.

CHAPTER FIVE

Creating the Guy's and St Thomas' NHS Trust, 1991-1999

Overview

The 1990s was a decade of tumultuous change triggered by the merger of Guy's and St Thomas' Trusts as part of the wider reconfiguration of London health services following the Tomlinson Review. Merging governance, management, and services of the two hospitals was a complex and acrimonious affair. Each hospital established campaign groups which battled to secure primacy for their respective sites as the merger unfolded. The emotional impacts of the changes were deeply felt by all staff, and the slow process of building a shared culture of care raised fundamental questions about professional identities and values. The decade also marked a milestone in the longer history of the medical and dental schools as UMDS merged with King's College London. By the approach of the new millennium, the merged Guy's and St Thomas' Trust was moving forwards and starting to reap some of the benefits for patients and services. The chapter closes by exploring how the new institutional identity was experienced by patients and staff against a backdrop of changing approaches to patient care and patients' emerging agency in the 1990s hospital system.

Reconfiguring London health services

The introduction of market mechanisms to the NHS opened the way for London purchasing authorities to look beyond the teaching hospitals which were some of the most expensive in the UK, to district general hospitals in outer London that offered much better value for money. This created significant risk to the teaching hospitals because if the flow of patients into London was reversed outwards, then patient numbers would fall below the requirements set for accredited specialist training by the Royal Colleges.[1] The King's Fund had set up its own enquiry into London healthcare in July 1990 with a focus on protecting the interests of London people in the context of the anticipated changes of the market, and William Waldegrave, Secretary of State for Health, commissioned a Government enquiry into London health services, medical education, and research in autumn 1991. Sir Bernard Tomlinson, who was a consultant pathologist in Newcastle-upon-Tyne and chair of the North East RHA, was appointed to head the enquiry with Terms of Reference set as advising on 'the provision of healthcare in inner London, working within the framework of the reformed NHS'.[2]

In April 1992 the Conservatives unexpectedly won the General Election under the leadership of John Major, and Virginia Bottomley replaced Waldegrave as Secretary of State for Health. Previously a junior minister in the Department of Health, Virginia had been instrumental in Bernard Tomlinson's appointment. Virginia also had close connections to St Thomas': her father, John Garnett, was chair of Lambeth District Health Authority between 1986 and 1990, and her daughter was studying medicine at UMDS in the early 1990s. In 2013 during a Witness Seminar, Virginia explained she originated from a 'medical mafia' and reflected on the challenges of inheriting the Tomlinson report. She was unequivocal that the scale of the London problem required action.

> I had told John Major I knew the report was coming up. I said, I will do the heavy lifting, the dirty stuff and then I can move off before the election. Perhaps not many people have my masochistic personality ... Why was I so stoical?

Partly because, up and down the country, everybody else was making these decisions…But on the other hand, I was not political. John Major had said, do you need help? I said, no, no, I'm fine. I'd always said, I'll do the dirty work and when I've done the dirty work, somebody else can take it on and be nice. In politics you have window-breakers and glaziers. I was the glazier in bedding in the NHS reforms that had got noisy for Ken Clarke, but I had to be the window-breaker on London change.[3]

Momentum built as the King's Fund published the results of their enquiry in June, and the following month the South East Thames RHA submitted a report to Tomlinson suggesting that either Guy's or St Thomas' Hospital should close.[4] In October Tomlinson published his recommendations which included reducing overall numbers of beds, moving funding from the acute to the primary sector, and closing/merging various of the London hospitals. In the South East Thames region, the report concluded, only three at most of the four major hospitals (King's, Guy's, Lewisham, and St Thomas') would be required in five years' time. King's and Lewisham were believed to have a 'secure' future as they had natural patient populations, and so Tomlinson recommended the creation of 'a single management structure for Guy's and St Thomas' with services rationalised on one site'. Guy's and Lewisham Trust were to split, with Lewisham continuing to operate as a standalone hospital. He also noted that 'our analysis shows St Thomas' to be slightly more vulnerable than Guy's particularly in the area of costs'.[5] The prospect of such significant change was intensely contested by all involved and emotions ran high. That Tomlinson did not state which site should close was not surprising: 'I think he ducked the issue, because it was a very, very difficult nettle to grasp,' reflected John Pelly, Finance Director at St Thomas'. *Making London Better*, the Government's formal response to the Tomlinson Report, was published in February 1993.[6] By that point Virginia had convened a small team to work with her including

Kenneth Calman, Chief Medical Officer, and Duncan Nichol, Chief Executive of the NHS, and former administrator at St Thomas'. The London Implementation Group (LIG) was set up with Tim Chessells, chairman of North East Thames RHA serving as chair, and Bob Nicholls, regional manager of Oxford RHA and former administrator at St Thomas', as Chief Executive Officer. The LIG launched specialty reviews of cardiac, cancer, renal and neuroscience services, and became a primary sounding board for the Government.[7]

Tim Chessells recalls being interviewed at length by Tomlinson and reviewing the draft report. He reflected that the haphazard location of hospitals in London resulted from a political culture in which 'no-one has ever had the courage to stop people doing things but give them half of it or a quarter of it or tell them they can have it later'. He elaborates:

> My own feeling about the underlying problem is that services grew up in a fairly haphazard fashion. All the teaching hospitals wanted to have expertise in every field. There was really no rational allocation of services, so that they were offering specialist services in quite small departments sometimes which are therefore very expensive to run. So inevitably they'd come up with financial problems and of course, the pressures on the health service, the aging population aren't new.[8]

The King's Fund and Tomlinson reports provided the LIG with a 'blueprint' to reduce the number of specialist services across London and strengthen those that remained. But although these policy directives guided decision-making, the LIG understood the importance of garnering support from staff and communities. Change was much easier to implement when clinicians and influential local figures, including MPs, advocated for reforms and promoted them based on improving quality of services and education.[9]

Reconfiguration of London services was driven by the anticipated impact of the internal market on London health services as well as the political pressures of an election.[10] Yet the Government's decision to invest financially in setting up Trusts across London so close to undertaking a major reconstruction of acute health services was extraordinary, noted Karen Caines, General Manager at Guy's and Lewisham Trust.

> Well, I mean people had been muttering around for years... too many hospitals in London...if you look at it, it's an extraordinary thing for a government to do, isn't it? If you think you're going to have major amalgamations of London hospitals, then do not invest large sums of money in setting up Trusts...in any rational world you wouldn't have done it. The Government could simply have said, until we've cleared the configuration of hospitals in London, no one's going to get Trust status. And then we'll take it from there. But they didn't. So, I think in some ways, it had been on the cards for a long time, and in other ways it came as a surprise...What came as a total surprise to me, and, I think, a completely muddle-headed piece of thinking, that in fact didn't materialise, was, the original proposition was one site...I think Tommy's were worried that Guy's had this flagship thing, and they wanted Guy's and Thomas' to work together, to see off King's. But King's does serve a local population and Guy's and Thomas', at the end of the day, it isn't quite a stone's throw, but they aren't that far away from each other. But the idea of wasting all that infrastructure, and just moving to a one-site solution, and neither site could have taken what was needed. Potty![11]

The London Health Emergency (LHE) campaign group (established in 1983) was swift to challenge the statistics underpinning the argument for reducing hospital bed capacity in the capital. The

Tomlinson Report estimated a surplus of between 2000 and 7000 beds owing to a reduction of inpatients from outside London and greater efficiency in bed use.[12] John Lister, Director of LHE, recollected the issues around inaccurate data.

> Tomlinson had been an extraordinary report…based pretty much in Central London and didn't really explore very much outside the peripheries. And so, you had a whole section of the map that missed off, you know, I think, it was Barking, Havering, and Brentwood were just missed off the Greater London map, and the hospitals out there and so forth. There were some classic errors, and some hospitals that were listed in there that weren't part of London at all, and various other things. So, we were able to make a bit of fun out of that. But they proposed a cut of something like 4,000 beds, and we pointed out this would be devastating to do this. And in the end, they also proposed to completely close a number of hospitals, so Guy's or Tommy's should have closed under the Tomlinson proposals. In the end, they merged them together and they kept the most of both of them, so I think, you know, we can't claim credit for all of that at all. But I mean, I think the fact that we were part of the pressure that made them consider whether they wanted to drive through the whole thing, they wanted to shut Barts, Barts is now part of this massive redevelopment in East London, and we managed to keep that. We held onto it until Labour got in, and Labour held onto it.[13]

The data was also challenged by Brian Jarman, Professor of Primary Care at St Mary's Hospital Medical School, who published his analysis of London bedding requirements in April 1993.[14]

> I did strongly oppose the closure of the hospitals mainly because I felt that the analysis that they'd done was utterly

incorrect, they'd actually got it completely the wrong way round… It didn't seem feasible that London had an excess of beds when we had, in the preceding few years to when this report started, had particular difficulties getting people admitted to hospital. I actually knew that there is a thing called the EBS, the emergency bed service, which is what we were using as GPs if we have difficulty getting a patient admitted to hospital. You could measure the usage of the need to EBS patient, and they were measured and what I did was to say to, I phoned up the Tomlinson Committee and I said, look you can get some information about whether London's over-bedded and has there have been any change 'cos there is the EBS data. You can look it up yourselves. And they did look it up and, in the Tomlinson Report they said, we've done this, and we've found there's a reduction in the use of EBS. Again, doesn't seem quite right so I looked at their data and the data had gone up I think three times the usage over the preceding four years or so and of course it went up in a sort of zigzag manner and just before the report came out there was a part where it had gone down 1.5 per cent and they had chosen that as the report they'd done. Again, what I felt was a manipulation of data rather than looking at the entire trend over a period of time which was obviously very sharply up over the preceding four years.[15]

Brian also alluded to the difficulties the Government experienced in getting data that was up to date and accurate.

I felt sorry for Virginia Bottomley who was the Secretary of State at the time because I was presenting her with information and data which we had in our department in masses, with the statisticians and the researchers to analyse it and the Department of Health doesn't do analyses. She was unable to have similar analyses herself to answer the questions that needed to be asked like the flows in mortality data. She just had to accept the things that had been given to her which, as I said earlier on, I felt had been skewed in a way to produce the answers that they wanted. But our data was all in the public domain; we published it, and anyone could look at it and no-one has ever questioned it.[16]

The Tomlinson recommendations produced a furore across London and as the changes began to be implemented, the reconfiguration of London health services remained prominent across health publications including *Hospital Doctor, Pulse, Health Services Journal*, national broadsheets, and local publishers including *South London Press* and *Health Emergency: Monthly Bulletin of London Health Emergency*.[17]

Setting up the new Trust Board

The absence of detailed recommendations within Tomlinson and from Whitehall on the siting of the merged trust and the rationalisation of services fostered ambiguity and speculation on the fate of each hospital. The process began in December 1992 with the appointment of Lord Barney Hayhoe, former Conservative MP and Minister for Health 1985-1986, to a non-executive role designed 'to give support during the period of consultation'.[18] Barney was established as the prospective Chairman of the new Trust in January 1993. Yet the other contender for chair, Philip Harris, former chair of Guy's and Lewisham Trust and major fundraiser for the Conservative Party, had appeared to many to be the strongest candidate. As one interviewee put it, Lord Harris was 'hands on' and Lord Hayhoe was 'hands off': 'if you walked round the hospital with Phil, it took a very long time because he knew every cleaner by name, every porter by name, he knew whether the cleaner had bunions, or the porter's mother was poorly. He was a real people person'.[19]

As Chair of the merged Trust, Lord Hayhoe headed the appointment panel in early March 1993 for the new chief executive for which there were two contenders: Peter Griffiths, Chief Executive of Guy's and Lewisham, and Tim Matthews, Chief Executive of St Thomas'. The widely-expressed expectation was that Peter Griffiths would be appointed. During a ministerial meeting on the day before the interview, Virginia Bottomley said to Duncan Nichol, NHS Chief Executive who was the assessor on the appointment, 'it's going to be all right tomorrow, isn't it, Duncan? Nod nod, wink wink, code to those of us in the know, that meant that the Guy's incumbent was going to get the job'.[20] In the event, Duncan Nichol did not attend the interview and the decision was made to appoint Tim: Victoria Bottomley was 'flaming mad and couldn't understand what had gone on'. The vote had been split and Lord Hayhoe had the casting vote. His decision to appoint Tim in favour of Peter Griffiths was perceived to relate not just to his closeness to St Thomas' but also to avoid the political difficulties of implementing Peter's widely-known view that the merger should take place on one site only which meant the closure of the other site. Tim, however, had led St Thomas' submission to the Tomlinson Enquiry which included proposals that Guy's A&E department should close; St Thomas' should develop as the major provider of local acute and emergency services; and Guy's should develop as a tertiary and specialist hospital.[21]

Interviewees who had been involved in the processes surrounding the appointments of chair and chief executive were frank about their beliefs that the decisions were moulded by political considerations. It is hard to overstate the devastating impact of Tim Matthews' appointment on Guy's staff. Even though subsequent Board appointments were more fairly divided between the institutions, Guy's community experienced a deep sense of grief and loss that permeated all merger proceedings.

It was like a bereavement, [Peter] was at that time the golden boy of the NHS, and everybody thought he was going to get the job…that started a really difficult period of time because everybody thought everybody at St Thomas's would get the jobs. There was actually a real sharing out of the jobs, but it was always going to be St Thomas's led.[22]

Tim Matthews was appointed…and he appointed his Finance Director, without interview and that's when everybody got the wind up, because they felt they were all going to be selected and there would be no interviews. And I think that was when it got quite tense and then it was agreed there would be two medical directors, the one from Guy's and the one from St Thomas', but all the other posts would be competitive. And then there was all the rumours, there wouldn't be assessors and the assessors would be chosen because they would…it was all very unpleasant.[23]

In hindsight, it is difficult to say whether this appointment did ultimately affect the outcomes.

I think it was very hard work for the St Thomas' chief executive they did appoint, a really big job in trying to bring the two cultures together. Now whether it would have gone any quicker or any better if it had gone the other way, who knows? You can't say. But it certainly wasn't what was expected and what the Secretary of State was expecting to happen. So even when you think things are being controlled quite carefully from the centre, they don't always turn out in the same way.[24]

Several interviewees reflected that the only way of avoiding such fallout would have been to have appointed from outside Guy's and St Thomas'.

What I'm about to say is no reflection on the Chief Executive who was appointed, or the Chief Executive who was not appointed from the two hospitals, but it was an error not to bring in an outsider who could not be perceived as being biased one way or the other. As I say this is no reflection on the actual appointment and it would have happened either way whoever had been appointed from Guy's or Thomas'. But it ensured a difficult ride for some years and in my view hampered the attempts at getting the two hospitals to work together.[25]

If somebody had seen the passions that were about to unfold, I think they could have been more sensible in appointing a neutral chairman and a mix across the board, that everybody could have looked up to.[26]

Peter Griffiths' sensemaking of the episode illuminates the way in which the opportunities for rationalisation of services were curtailed by the political constraints at the time.

It was clear, quite understandably, that Virginia Bottomley and Lord Hayhoe and the new board did not want to see, did not expect to see, any significant rationalisation of services really between Guy's and Thomas'. They expected to see one management, but they certainly wanted to move away from the proposition that one or other site would prevail, and to have a more collaborative approach to their future together. I can certainly see why that occurred and why that would have been their motivation...I think those of us associated with Guy's were seen as too controversial and too high profile and this was an opportunity for changing that. I suspect I'd have taken that view if I had been them... essentially we thought that what was happening at the time was the opportunity through merger to make serious rationalisation of services and to become seriously more efficient, and we misjudged that…certainly my leadership at Guy's, certainly Phil Harris's leadership at Guy's, and what might happen if we had become leaders of Guy's and Thomas', would have been regarded as very risky because we would have, as I say, wanted to have made significant changes and may even have wanted to close one of the hospitals. I think some people thought that if we had have been put in leadership positions, we may have tried to do that in quite an aggressive way whereas what was perceived, I think, behind the scenes as being required, was a period of peace and tranquillity, not a period of further major hassle. Now that's an irony given that the whole notion of the Tomlinson report for London was to bring about significant rationalisation of services in London. As I said, it never resulted in doing that. It brought about a rationalisation of management of hospitals in London, which is not at all the same thing. So, my simple take on it is that I don't think the Secretary of State and politicians were serious about rationalisation.[27]

The new Trust Board appointments were made by the end of March 1993 and included five non-executive directors: Professor Cyril Chantler (UMDS), Nigel Clark (Head of Personnel, ICI), Tim Ford (Partner, Park Nelson Solicitors), Victoria Silvester (Home Economics Consultant), and Clive Williams (Managing Partner, Ernst and Young). The five executive directors were: Tim Matthews, Chief Executive (St Thomas'); John Pelly, Director of Finance (St Thomas'); Wilma MacPherson, Nursing Director (Guy's); Karen Caines, Project Director (Guy's); and Tony Young (St Thomas') and Professor Michael Maisey (Guy's), joint Medical Directors.[28] The new Trust became fully operational on 1 April 1993. An immediate visible commitment to fairness between the two hospitals was made at the outset through Tim Matthews and Karen Caines swopping their offices. Both were beautiful offices, but Karen conceded that the view of the river at St Thomas' had much to commend it. Another early and easy decision was the name of the merged Trust.

> We had the discussion very early on in the board and we said, St Thomas' and Guy's, Guy's and St Thomas'. Guy's and St Thomas' just sounds better, doesn't it? Everybody agreed. It just sounds better and that was as simple as that.[29]

The Board came together to work in good faith but 'in the community at large, it was horrendous, people who did clearly not like each other, to the point of most extraordinary behaviour. And there was a hell of a lot of institutional gameplay!'.

> There had always been a degree of tribal animosity between [Guy's and St Thomas'] …I might lose my job wasn't the biggest anxiety. I think it was just…don't like them, don't want to merge with them. Bizarre. And in some cases when it actually came to merger, really just vicious and unpleasant. Quite weirdly so actually. A psychiatrist would have had a field day.[30]

The mandate from Virginia Bottomley made it clear that the Board's initial task was to decide which hospital should close and several interviewees affirmed that the outcome about sites was not circumscribed by Virginia or the Department of Health. But no one could imagine that any government would be willing to take the political fallout of closing St Thomas' with its iconic position opposite the Houses of Parliament and status as the designated hospital for visiting heads of state. Interestingly, internal government documents suggest that there was a Department-held view that 'there would be a single NHS site at Guy's'.[31] The assumption that the merger would involve the closure on one hospital site 'almost institutionalised that tribal defensiveness from the start' reflected Tim Matthews, adding 'when you're trying to build a sense of unity and a mission and a vision for a new organisation and you know one of you is going to close that made life incredibly more difficult than it needed to be'. Amidst uncertainties about the closure of sites, reorganisation of services, and fears of redundancies, and the furore across London about the various reconfigurations, the campaign movements in both hospitals ramped up their efforts to ensure their site was prioritised.

Save Guy's Hospital campaign

As the 'flagship' Trust with innovative management, a strong research portfolio and the ongoing development of the Phase III capital investment programme, Guy's was reasonably confident at the outset that its site would be favoured in the merger. But the failure of Peter Griffiths to secure the post of chief executive caused extreme alarm across the Guy's community and the campaigning intensified. Staff from all parts of Guy's joined in and this reinforced the sense of the institution being a family with tight bonds that cross-cut roles and levels of seniority.

> Consultants led the battle, they were people who'd trained there, and they'd lived their lives there. Bob Knight, who was one of the great consultant leaders, Mike Gleeson, Steve Challacombe, pretty well every professor in every department became involved in the campaigns, and lots of doctors and lots of nurses were involved in the Save Guy's campaign, and lots of radiographers, I mean at all levels the Guy's family was really strong, the wives of the consultants, some of the other female members of staff were the volunteers all the time in the office.[32]

Richard Hughes, consultant neurologist, had trained in Guy's in the early 1960s and was the third generation of his family to do so. Bob Knight asked him to chair the committee which met once a week.

We used to compare notes with each other about the different developments and try to collect the evidence on which we could build a case for the Accident and Emergency department being placed at Guy's rather than at St Thomas' Hospital. Evidence like transport links, for instance, which actually are much better to Guy's rather than St Thomas'…we produced a number of documents.[33]

Betsy Morley, a Guy's nursing school alumnus and senior site nursing manager who had worked there from 1988, was an active member. She described how the merger was perceived as the end of Guy's with all staff experiencing a strong sense of loss: 'right from consultant level right down, everybody was very depressed about the demise…I think the decision had been made, to be honest, however hard we tried. All the staff felt that we were losing Guy's as it were'.[34] Stalwart campaigners like Professor Michael Gleeson maintained his strong views that the merger 'was a stitch up. It was a takeover'.[35]

Guy's local community rallied against the hospital's potential closure through the 'Save It Casualty Crisis' (SICC) Campaign. Malcolm Alexander, whose role as chief officer at Camberwell (later Southwark) Community Health Council included oversight of safety at Guy's and St Thomas', was involved in monitoring the emergency services at London hospitals.

We went round carrying sick buckets to collect resources for the campaign. And we had a SICC shop in Bermondsey… the SICC campaign was the community campaign, and the Save Guy's campaign was the campaign led by consultants. And we kind of, under the auspices of the Community Health Council (CHC), we gradually joined those together and we supported, with CHC resources, the Save Guy's campaign. We were under the impression that we had saved Guy's from closing. And I say that because the original plan was to close it completely. And we took a number of measures, including marches, demonstrations, blocking traffic just by the Rotherhithe Tunnel, taking a judicial review, and many other activities to stop Guy's from closing.[36]

The shared priority of campaigning to save Guy's from closure enabled a strong alliance to be forged across hospital and community groups. Guy's was a focal point for civic pride and was embedded in the community. Simon Hughes, Liberal Democrat MP who was a key player in the campaign, explained the meaning of Guy's for Bermondsey people and the significance of Guy's Tower, opened in 1974, for the local landscape.

> Guy's was our big local hospital, obviously there were smaller hospitals in those days, now gone, St Olave's Hospital in Rotherhithe, St Giles in Camberwell, there was the Lambeth Hospital, but Guy's was the local hospital and everybody saw it as the hospital for Bermondsey...it was visibly part of the community because of its rather ugly but very tall tower building, it was much loved by the community, and it was hugely regarded by the community as a centre of excellence.[37]

The Guy's campaign highlighted the natural advantages offered by Guy's compared to St Thomas' producing Fact Sheets that evidenced how the Guy's site was 60,000 square metres greater than St Thomas', the location was closely attached to multiple transport routes, and it offered high-quality facilities including the new Philip Harris House. Moreover, its record of scientific research was measurably higher in terms of external grant funding and publications. Maurice Lessof emphasised the comparative accessibility of Guy's for South East London patients.[38] Simon Hughes noted 'in terms of people getting in and out because London Bridge Station was next to the hospital, and literally next to it in a way Waterloo isn't to St Thomas's, then Guy's was an obvious location to keep as the main hospital'.[39]

Political support for Guy's came from across the spectrum including Simon Hughes MP and other prominent political supporters like Labour MP Harriet Harman. Kay Lucey, an auxiliary nurse, provides an insight into how the plight of saving Guy's became a political issue. Her memory reveals the spectre of Thatcher in proceedings, and how Labour worked with the campaign whilst in opposition.

> Margaret Thatcher started shutting Guy's down. I was involved in that with the union because basically we had to go to Simon Hughes, who was the local MP. He was marvellous, I mean he went to Parliament, he brought it up in Parliament and Tony Blair (Labour leader from 1994) was looking to get in that time and came to Guy's, so we'd vote him in and all that. And he promised to keep Guy's Hospital open and of course, he went back on that the minute he got in.[40]

Professor Michael Gleeson also noted how the support that came from Labour whilst they were in opposition waned once Labour gained office in 1997: 'they were very grateful for us helping them get rid of the Major Government but of course, they did little more'.[41] There were also personal links between the Department of Health and Guy's. Surgeon Ian McColl, for example, had a strong relationship with John Major, becoming his Parliamentary Private Secretary in 1994. Despite these factors, Guy's perceived St Thomas' to have stronger and tighter political connections and the benefits of a bias from the establishment. Simon Hughes MP reflected on how this coloured the Guy's campaign.

> St Thomas's was directly opposite the Palace of Westminster, and it was terribly convenient as a hospital for

Parliamentarians, for Ministers, and for the Civil Servants including in the Department of Health. So, we knew we were confronted with a competitor, as it were, to become the sole hospital, which would have a lot of backers. I also think I remember correctly that Virginia Bottomley may even have done some training at Tommy's and her daughter was a medic there, and so there were various reasons why people thought there might be an establishment favouritism towards Tommy's which we knew was a battle we'd have to deal with.[42]

Notwithstanding the kudos of being the flagship Trust and the demonstrable success in cutting costs whilst improving services between 1991 and 1993, the failure of Guy's leaders to secure the appointment of chair or chief executive created deep distrust of the way in which decisions about the reconfiguration of services across the sites would be made. Guy's staff in leadership positions found themselves working in a confrontational atmosphere and Wilma MacPherson, Director of Nursing, reflected that her long connections with the institution were disregarded.

It was very hard. I mean, I was labelled a traitor. I'd been about a year and a half there in total, and because I wasn't heading the Guy's campaign, I was sort of really ostracised by colleagues, medical colleagues particularly, who I'd known for a long time. But I mean, it was something I obviously couldn't do. And apart from that, I didn't feel it was the right thing to do. But if I had, I would have had to have given up my job. So, it was not a good time.[43]

Save St Thomas' Hospital campaign

At St Thomas', the Tomlinson report and the imposed merger with Guy's changed the new Trust's agenda 'quite dramatically', reflected

Tim Matthews. Rather than forging ahead as an independent institution the key question focused on how St Thomas' could position itself as being of 'equal strength' to Guy's as the merger processes began.

> Guy's had very successfully positioned itself as the flagship NHS Trust, was flying the flag for Trust status and had a very high profile in doing so. St Thomas' conversely had been through a period of quite significant and quite public financial difficulties and was perceived potentially as being the weaker partner. So, to put it crudely, there was real sense that we needed to get our shit together, you know, if we weren't going to be swamped by the ravaging hordes coming down from Bermondsey![44]

Sir Robert Reid, chair of St Thomas' had 'accepted' the need for the rationalisation of hospital care across London before the Tomlinson review but was of the view that St Thomas' should be 'robust in defending ourselves against hostile attacks. This we managed to achieve by providing excellent results backed by good communications'.[45] At no point in its long history had St Thomas' perceived itself to be the underdog in any context and this gave rise to the 'feeling around the hospital that we were, kind of, manning the barricades'.[46] It generated a vigorous and comprehensive response from consultants and managers which took the form of a three-strand strategy: demonstrating robust financial health; a vigorous marketing campaign with key influencers to get the St Thomas' 'brand' better known; and building a strong, analytical rationale for why St Thomas' needed to be retained as an acute hospital with an Accident and Emergency department. The appointment of Tim Bell, public relations expert, and confidante of Margaret Thatcher to advise on communications strategy was funded by the endowment funds, and although the move was heavily criticised, it paid dividends in shifting public perceptions of St Thomas' as vulnerable to closure to being a strong contender in the context of the merger. The strength of the data that was produced sought to provide rational arguments for difficult choices about site reconfigurations.

> We weren't just doing that to defend the indefensible and I think that the strength of what we did and which came through ultimately was, you know, our positioning wasn't based on, you know, save this institution, it was based on some very detailed much, much better analysis I think, you know, it wasn't done by me, but that had been done anywhere else in London about the pattern and distribution of particularly emergency services...Bob O'Leary did all of this work and produced isochrone maps which mapped in much more detail than anybody else was doing, the potential impact of service change on different population groups and people's access, you know, and travel times to work.[47]

Colonel Malcolm Ross, Comptroller of the Lord Chamberlain's office, responsible for the Queen's Medical Household, apparently expressed concerns in a letter: 'St Thomas' is the central hospital for state events. I cannot emphasise too strongly the importance we attach to this, and I hope an outcome will be found which will permit it to remain so.'[48] Several interviewees dismissed as irrelevant the notion that St Thomas' political and establishment connections were instrumental in terms of outcomes.

> Basically, we had tended to provide, not always, the surgeon to the Royal household and the physician to the Royal household. Nothing really. It was about as meaningless as the masonic thing, which still amazes me when I think about it. But it's the sort of thing when you're looking round for some kind of reason other than rationality for why things turned out the way they did you're going to

conjure up all sorts of reasons: oh, they're all public-school boys, they've all got the Royal family in their pockets, and they're all masons.[49]

Yet it was and remains impossible to imagine the Houses of Parliament and the Palace of Westminster being onlookers to the repurposing of the St Thomas' site if it were to close.

John Lister, then Director of London Health Emergency, recalls the differing approach at St Thomas', noting the lack of TUC union activism there and the more significant role played by the Royal College of Nursing.

> The Royal College of Nursing has always been much stronger, relatively, in St Thomas' than, you know, the unions we deal with are TUC unions primarily. In fact, we've never been able to campaign with the RCN, they've never done anything that's related to London Health Emergency.[50]

The Staff Side at St Thomas' which was the interface between the professional bodies like the RCN, the unions, and the organisation, was deeply involved in the campaign. In December 1992, Kate Hoey, Labour MP for Vauxhall, joined doctors on a barge on the Thames whilst hundreds of nurses joined hands and stretched from St Thomas' across Westminster Bridge to the Houses of Parliament. Protest flags saying 'Save St Thomas' Hospital' were flown from the boat, remembered Marianne Vennegoor, dietician and chair of the Staff Side.[51]

Siting of the A&E

Tomlinson had recommended consolidating services on one site and John Pelly, finance director, explained how from a cost perspective, closing one site would produce savings.

Fundamentally, Guy's and St Thomas' are physically a mile
and a half apart and there was clearly a lot of duplication of
services and therefore a lot of excess cost that, on the face
of it, could be driven out if one or other were to close or at
least if parts of one or other were to close.[52]

But the new Trust Board realised very quickly that the only way to
move forwards as a single organisation was to remove the threat of
closure by proposing a dual-site solution. 'If we can at least allay
a proportion of this sense of threat then we might at least start
moving some of the way forward and people might see more in it
for them and their service than they do of defending their patch.'[53]
A range of options was formally reviewed including single and split
site configurations.[54]

We increasingly built the strategy around, how can you
optimise a twin site solution, which meets the financial
targets that we've been set? So demonstrates that for
financial reasons, we don't need to amalgamate all services
onto one site and, indeed, to do so, would be horrendously
expensive in capital terms, but, at the same time, develop
a solution and a strategy which delivers major change,
which facilitates the rationalisation of departments, creates
opportunities for academic growth, etc, etc, but using the
sites in a radically different way. There was a huge amount
of toing and froing that the twin medical directors, at the
time, were involved in, in leading about, both how you did
that. What was the most sensible distribution of services,
recognising that there was always going to be rough ends
that you couldn't perfectly map, particularly given that you
had to work, to a very large degree, with the grain of the
physical fabric that we had, and we had limited opportunity
for real capital investment. The Government said to us,
you've got £100m, it sounds a lot of money, but does not go

hugely far in reorganising a place like Guy's and Thomas'
over the whole lifecycle of this change.[55]

By December 1993, the Trust Board had determined that the most
effective strategy was to develop St Thomas' as an acute general
hospital – the hot site – and Guy's as a leading tertiary care centre –
the cold site. They concluded that a single site option would be the
'least flexible' and would also require major capital investment.[56] The
LIG independently assessed the business case and concluded that it
'carries significant clinical disadvantages and generates high revenue
costs because of split site working'.[57] The Trust was asked to appraise
further options which considered the ongoing merger between
UMDS and King's College and the siting of the merged schools
and departments. The appraisal was returned to the Department
'without [the Trust] making any further recommendations on a
preferred option'.[58] The Department of Health's final decision ran to
the wire. On 31 January 1994 Virginia Bottomley's principal private
secretary sent briefing notes to the Treasury.

> A note on the issues affecting Guy's and St Thomas' –
> here the health and education interests are still pulling in
> different directions. The decisions are extremely finely-
> balanced and commonsense does not indicate an obvious
> solution. Problems of leadership have contributed to the
> tensions in the institution.[59]

In one of the meetings that took place with the LIG and Department
officials, Virginia Bottomley called in a group of UMDS medical
students, one of whom was her daughter, to ask their opinion about
the siting of the medical school.

> I can remember a famous meeting in the Secretary of State's
> office when we were still wrestling about which should be
> the hot site. The Secretary of State called in some medical

students from UMDS to seek their opinion. Consulting the next generation, I think, she called it. One of them was her daughter, who was a medical student at UMDS at the time. I can remember it very clearly to this day. They were surprised they were being asked the question because they said, well St Thomas' is an absolutely useless site for students. There's no pubs, facilities, social arrangements, and Guy's already has a fair amount of academic space and development and is a much better social centre for students to be at and so we should develop that as the academic centre. So that meant the hot site should be St Thomas'.[60]

A 31 January 1994 draft of the Ministerial Statement on the implementation of the Tomlinson changes still contained blanks in the section referring to Guy's and St Thomas' where the specific hospital sites were referenced.[61] But on 10 February 1994, Virginia Bottomley announced to the House of Commons that the decision had been taken to locate the A&E on the St Thomas' site.

> The St Thomas's site offers a better location and environment for a hospital and serves a bigger local population. The need to safeguard what is the largest and one of the busiest accident and emergency departments in London was also crucial to the decision. We therefore intend to ask the Trust to pursue proposals that, over time, will concentrate acute and specialist hospital services at the St Thomas's site. As well as clinical teaching accommodation, a strong research presence, in conjunction with acute clinical services, will be retained on the St Thomas's site. Under these proposals, the Guy's site would offer a wide range of modern hospital and health services focused on the needs of the local community. [Guy's] accident and emergency department would remain at the site until alternative facilities were developed and were working satisfactorily.[62]

The decision over the siting of the A&E was the most difficult of the whole merger. At the time of the merger St Thomas' had just completed Phase 1 of a £3.25 million expansion of their A&E department, prompted by the closure of the Westminster Hospital causing an increase in patient numbers, and estimates were for 100,000 attendances a year.[63] Richard Hughes described the importance of the A&E to the sense of what a hospital was.

> We saw the accident and emergency department as being the lifeblood of a proper hospital and that you couldn't be a proper hospital without an accident and emergency department. And if you had an accident and emergency department, you had to have the main specialties on that site; you had to have medicine, you had to have surgery, you had to have paediatrics, you had to have obstetrics and gynaecology. And we felt that we would become a lesser hospital without one.

The A&E was 'always the sort of outward and visible sign of a major local hospital', explained MP Simon Hughes and thus had strong symbolic meaning.[64] Consultant Jangu Banatvala put it more bluntly: 'if you lose your A&E department it does to some extent emasculate you'.[65] The combination of good patient access and facilities available at Guy's had led staff to hope that they would secure the A&E.

> We hoped we would get the acute because we felt that it was easier to get to Guy's for people coming…a lot of our patients came up from the south for specialist care, cardiology, renal. We had a big renal unit, a big kids' unit, much bigger than St Thomas', and a new paediatric intensive care. So, we were quite confident that we would get the acute, because we'd been told that between the two hospitals there would be one that would be taking the acute

work and one that would be less acute and concentrating more on a campus for the students.[66]

The decision was highly contested. Southwark Community Health Council, MP Simon Hughes, and the Save Guy's campaign applied to seek a judicial review on the basis that they had been 'blatantly denied' the right to full consultations over the decision to move A&E services to St Thomas'. But the application was refused by Mr Justice Laws on the basis that there had been too long a delay in launching the challenge.[67] The political backlash was significant, with Conservative MPs losing faith in Virginia Bottomley's reforms – the planned closure of St Bartholomew's and Guy's A&E were the most prominent examples of London institutions served the 'death warrant' by the health minister.[68] 'I had to go through quite a process of vilification which is not enjoyable for anybody and for somebody who was in fact so personally committed to the cause as I was, it was I suppose a bit harsh,' Virginia later reflected.[69] The Save Guy's campaign continued to challenge the closure of the A&E with Simon Hughes MP giving strong support by raising the matter regularly in parliamentary debates and urging that the decision be reconsidered on the basis of the unprecedented rise in A&E attendances which would result in St Thomas' being expected to cope with more than double the number of attendances it was designed to take.[70] Despite assurances from New Labour before the 1997 general election that they would support Guy's, the announcement that Guy's A&E would finally close in 1999 was made by the new Labour Secretary of Health, Frank Dobson.[71]

In retrospect there is broad agreement that the decision played out well for both Guy's and St Thomas'.

It was a very short and intensive discussion and battle, and some would say, well, St. Thomas' won. Well, I'd say, no they didn't win…for the merged Guy's and Thomas' it was probably a very sound decision which actually later helped them establish a very viable complete range of services from district right through to specialty services.[72]

A very sensible compromise and it built on the academic strengths at Guy's, and Guy's became the academic campus and St Thomas' became the acute clinical campus, and a very good one, too. And some of the elective services were retained or built up on the Guy's campus, and that was very sensible.[73]

Locating the A&E on the St Thomas' site shaped the split of services and facilities across the two sites with trauma and urgent, non-elective treatment centred at St Thomas' with elective outpatient and academic facilities earmarked for investment at Guy's.[74]

Merging services

The emotional and psychological impact on staff from merging services and facilities was enormous. It is no surprise that Chairman Lord Barney Hayhoe was minded to issue a plea to: 'stop the in-fighting. The sooner we can make people understand that there is no going back, the sooner we can devote the whole energies of the Trust to the betterment of healthcare and prevention for the local population'.[75] Mike Maisey, Professor of Radiological Science at Guy's and joint Medical Director of the new Trust reflected on the intensity of feelings.

The thing that shocked me was not the level of antagonism but the intense hatred that some people had for other people. I think it shocked Tony [Young] and it shocked me. People used to come to see me and see him and express their feelings in the most outrageous language about colleagues in the other trust, their opposite numbers, and others, not only in their own specialty but also the whole concept of it. The sheer vitriol that was swilling around there made it extremely difficult for a lot of people to work and I don't think that should be underestimated. The other thing that surprised me was that this wasn't the older members of the staff entirely, it was as much the younger members of staff, some of whom hadn't even qualified at either Guy's or St Thomas'.[76]

The realisation that it was probably going to take ten years or so to move beyond the 'grief and blood' and achieve harmony across the organisation led Karen Caines who had spear-headed the development of the merged Trust's plan, to leave.

I genuinely did not want to spend the precious years of my life in this kind of heart-breaking institutional wrangle. There are better things to do than that. And I wasn't really committed to either side, in a sense, I could move on without it being any great difficulty to me.

Carole Rowe had worked as a haematologist at Guy's since she left school in 1979 and loved the buzz of the hospital, describing herself as 'privileged' to work there. But from 1990 as Guy's began to lose its identity as a single hospital, she remembers things changing significantly.

Before it was a joy to go into work. You'd laugh from nine o'clock to five o'clock whereas [from 1990] the work got tougher, there was more paperwork and there wasn't the camaraderie there. It was just a case of churning out blood counts. The laughter and the happiness dropped away.

During the same period, Carole's mother became ill with cancer and as they wanted to move out of London, Carole found a job in Exeter Hospital.[77]

For clinicians, much of the antagonism was driven by the ways in which the merger cut across pre-existing long-term plans for service development. Michael Gleeson, senior lecturer from 1987 and later professor of medicine at UMDS, had established a specialist Ear, Nose and Throat (ENT) service at Guy's. He describes the struggle to retain the quality of the service in the context of the merger.

> I'd just spent seven or eight years planning a brand-new ENT department and got the money to equip it. It was probably the best-equipped ENT department in the country at the time. Microscopes on every unit and everything…We had the foresight to actually build the thing about three times as big as we actually needed at the time. Then my role in the Save Guy's campaign made it difficult for the Government to actually hit me personally because I had a profile, and they were scared to upset me, so they were not going to shut the ENT department at Guy's. They prevented me having my ward immediately next to my outpatient department, but I saved the most important bit, which was the outpatient department. I went through several years when St Thomas' tried to actually sell the building. They tried to put my department in the basement and cut its size to 30 per cent of what it was at a time when their own department was nothing more than a couple of tables with tablecloths on and a few assorted instruments. So, I did preserve that. I'm glad I did. I was absolutely right.[78]

Michael frames his fight for ENT in terms of St Thomas' staff attempting to overwhelm his service, in confrontation with management's designs for the merger. The intensity of feeling also led to some clinicians changing their referral patterns to avoid sending patients to clinicians they now regarded as enemies.

Wyndham Lloyd-Davies, consultant urologist at St Thomas', reflected on the way in which the merger also facilitated some clinical developments.

> Some very good decisions were made in the merger, I mean, urology being, in my view, one of the very, very best decisions that was made to create that really superb new unit at Guy's. And it was very difficult doing it across the two sites, because there was very much a partisan feeling of the two departments at the time. I became clinical director of the two, and it was very difficult to reconcile the situation, but the thing that healed the wound was that we had developed lithotripsy (a non-invasive technique for treating kidney stones) on the site and then it was taken into this wonderful new department, and it just brought everything together. It was a marvellous decision.[79]

The renal units providing dialysis and transplantation services for patients with chronic kidney disease were one of the first services to be merged and the new unit was sited at Guy's. At St Thomas', the service had been in an old building so even though it had good technology and high levels of staffing, the lift was often out of order and patients had then to walk up the stairs to the second floor. In contrast, Guy's unit seemed 'more welcoming, modern, fresher'.[80] Before the merger, clinical staff had had very little contact with each other although the technicians had formed networks through the Association of Renal Technicians which had been established in 1975. The consultant lead at the St Thomas' renal unit 'would not step foot on Guy's campus' which left the rest of the staff to carry on as best they could, trying to 'make things work and make things happen'.[81] In terms of services provided, the key difference was that St Thomas' had a smaller number of dialysis patients and ran a morning and afternoon shift, closing by six o'clock in the evening. Guy's was three times larger and ran an additional overnight shift. Staff perceived that there were sharp differences in the ways that care was delivered. At St Thomas', patients were known by name and the lower turnover gave nurses the time 'to be talkative and friendly'; Guy's had 'more of a business-like attitude'.[82] That some of these nuances were determined by work pressures rather than culture seems likely as after the units merged and satellite units were set up for dialysis in the community, the 'camaraderie' of the St Thomas' unit extended to Guy's staff as well.[83]

But the real rub of the tension was that 'we had totally different attitudes to work…there was a lot of animosity' and this played out most strongly in critiques of care.[84] St Thomas' was distinctive for having had a dietician as a clinical member of the renal team since the unit was set up in 1968. Patients with renal failure were not able to tolerate normal or high levels of protein and needed to keep low levels of sodium and phosphorus. Diet therefore played a critical role in maintaining health. When patients attended clinics, dietary advice and guidance was a core part of the service; in-patients had special menu cards tailored to their requirements. At Guy's, 'nutrition was just not on their list of priorities'.[85]

> It was a very sad time because I remember going to the renal unit in Guy's…patients were given cheese sandwiches and all kinds of sandwiches, and they should not have that food. So, I then talked to the nurses about it, and they said, well it's dialysed out, and, of course, it's not dialysed out, not phosphates, potassium yes, but not phosphate – that is actually dependent on the length of the dialysis treatment you are getting.[86]

Guy's criticisms of St Thomas' focused on the use of criteria for making difficult decisions about prioritising patients for treatment. Once dialysis and transplantation became established in the 1960s, many more patients required dialysis than there were resources available. Clinicians were left to develop a set of decision-making processes about which patients should be prioritised for treatment and this was common practice across the NHS. The clinical condition of the patients played a part but was by no means the most important factor. Other aspects such as the patient's contribution to society, their ability to commit to a strict diet and treatment regime, and family support networks all fed into the process. Guy's practice of treating all patients, regardless of age or circumstance, was felt to provide a very different quality of care.

> We had a perception that we put the patients first and that other renal units didn't, and that certainly, St Thomas' didn't...Guy's always did children, Guy's always did geriatrics...We didn't say because the patient was over 50 they wouldn't get treated, or they'd go to the back of the list...what we prided ourselves on was...we didn't have the restriction of saying we're not going to treat patients, based on status or points, or anything else.[87]

Interestingly despite the pressures on funding, dialysis became much more widely available by the late 1990s.

> When I first came to St Thomas' in '86, there was an age limit to what age they would treat people. If you was above a certain age, they wouldn't dialyse you, they said, no, no, we'll give priority to young people or people below that age. But now, it seems because of the patient's choice and the way the Health Service has moved on, everybody and anybody will be dialysed now. I've noticed we've got a lot of patients of an elderly age who are now being dialysed. When I first started, there wasn't a lot of renal spaces available for people, so they had to prioritise who got treated.[88]

It is difficult to retrospectively assess the accuracy of these claims and certainly the hospitals had different patient populations. The key point is that the distinctions drawn illustrate strongly how patient care in each hospital was imbued with specific philosophies that shaped staff identity and beliefs about the value of the work. Similar examples of interviewees expressing their discomfort through differences in the specificities of patient care in each institution are found in other examples of service mergers including the Intensive Care Units (ICU).

The merger of ICUs was highly acrimonious at the outset and the two Guy's consultant leads, David Bihari and Mark Smithies, resigned around the time of the announcement of the siting of the A&E. In a letter to the *Evening Standard*, David Bihari described the merger as a 'form of ethnic cleansing'.[89] The advantage of replacing consultants at this point was that the younger staff were able to see that the merger, although very unsettling, was also a time of opportunity for professional and organisational advancement. Merging services brought into question the differing styles of clinical practice that were of enormous importance in determining patient care, the skill make-up of teams, and shaping everyday routines. The merger of the ICUs was achieved through a formal process improvement project through which doctors and nurses sat down together to discuss practice and decide how things should be done as a merged team: 'that was surprisingly successful actually', remembered one clinician.[90] The consultants paired up so that each unit was headed by people from both hospitals, and this supported the integration: 'seeing ourselves as one new team'. One of the key differences between the ICUs was the specialisms and training of consultant staff. At Guy's, the clinicians were rooted in anaesthesia whereas at St Thomas', the clinicians originated from respiratory medicine: 'so we looked rather different in terms of how we had trained and come up the system'. These differences played out into clinical practice. At Guy's, patient care was closely aligned to research so patients were managed invasively with a lot of data collected and measurement of outcomes being done so that good care could be demonstrated. At St Thomas', clinical skills were understood as the driver for delivering the best care for patients and invasive procedures were avoided where possible. Over time, the integration of the two distinct clinical cultures enabled many positive aspects including the expansion in consultant specialisms to include nephrology as well as anaesthesia and respiratory medicine, and a shift in approaches to patient care to achieve: 'a rather happy midpoint now where they're probably more invasive than they used to be. We're probably less invasive because we've moved on with the advances in technology'.[91] In 2011 the merged ICU was one of six nationally commissioned centres to provide adult respiratory extracorporeal membrane oxygenation (ECMO) support.

Not surprisingly, out of all the groups involved in the merger, the consultants were the most intransigent about service change despite the strong and positive leadership from the Board and the clinical directors. The degree of tribalism between the two hospitals protracted the resolution of clinical issues during the merger, reflected one interviewee.[92] The Save Guy's campaign continued to lobby for a more equitable split of services across sites that foregrounded patient needs.[93] The strong resistance of clinicians to integrating services led to nurse leaders like Betsy Morley playing an essential peace-making role.

> We should all of us as nursing officers, both on the Thomas' and Guy's side, be proud of the fact that it was the nursing officers that made the way smooth to the merger. The consultants...some of them, particularly the surgeons, were, "well, certainly I'm not going to do it, I'm not doing whatever...I'm not going over there and so on". Laying down the law and saying what they would do, because

many of them were the old school. But the nursing officers, we had been told by Wilma, and she did a great job there, she got us all together and she said that we were the people who could ease the sufferings to the unhappiness between the two big hospitals by showing that we would make it work. I do think that happened. We got to know each other and yes, I think that was good.[94]

Every part of hospital life was impacted by the merger, including chaplaincy services. Guy's hospital chaplain, Neville Smith, described the merger as literally changing the shape of the organisation within which he worked.

One of the things that completely threw me in my last couple of years was the shape of the hospital changed when it really became Guy's and Thomas', because I always used to feel the hospital was triangular in shape, so you got the house governor at the top and spreading out and down, and then the auxiliary staff somewhere down at the...it's not very PC to put it this way, but it was that kind of...and I always felt that the chaplain, who was a bit outside this triangle, could actually slot into it at any given point. So, one moment you'd be talking to the house governor or the top person, and the next you'd be talking to Joe or whoever it was who wanted to come and mend your lock because you'd lost your keys or something like that, and you could ring up without filling in a form. So, it was very much an integrated kind of structure. Then it became building blocks. So, you got the medical, you got orthopaedics, you got paediatrics, and I couldn't slot in, and I didn't know how I was going to address these different building blocks. I had no place in any of them. Whereas in a triangular structure I had.[95]

In retrospect, across the interviews, there is broad consensus that the outcomes of the merger have been positive. But there is less concord that the management of the merger itself was managed as well as it could have been given the circumstances. One interesting aspect is that clinicians tend to remain more critical of the merger, than those who had held managerial roles and had been more directly invested in ensuring the success of the reforms.

> It's fair to say that there were consultants on both sides actually who felt very strongly that this was the wrong thing to do and that their institution was superior to the other, and so on, but in the event, the merger went well and Guy's and St Thomas' has gone on to be very, very successful in pretty much every respect in the ensuing years...I think that one of the keys was to appoint a clinical director for each of our major services encompassing both sites, which meant that they had to think about how best to organise that service across the sites.[96]

Some interviewees took solace from the fact that the Guy's and St Thomas' merger was more benign than others across London. The merger of their London counterparts – St Bartholomew's and The Royal London – for example, was described as 'a poisonous affair from the start'.[97] Whilst the wider institutional memory presents the merger as less vicious than other London hospitals, for individuals faced with animosity, particularly at Guy's, the amalgamation was an incredibly stressful period. Tony Young, joint and then sole Medical Director at Guy's and St Thomas', reflected on the merger in *The Medical Manager*, a practical guide for clinicians, first published in 1999, describing it as 'agonisingly difficult'.

> There was no very obvious winner and loser, both organisations won something, and both lost something; but Guy's perceived itself as the loser and the delicacy

of the equation goaded many people working within the organisation to subvert the process of the merger in larger or small ways. Whether that was an admirable commitment to a different vision or just short-sighted cussedness is a matter of opinion, but it certainly helped no one in the long term except some politicians … it was only in the midst of the Guy's and St Thomas' merger that I came to realise how like a death it seemed for many at Guy's, how important is the management of grieving, and how important it is to understand that the behaviour of some was akin to that of those close to a dying person: inappropriately focused anger, denial, and inability to function effectively. The arrangement of a merger between departments or hospitals taps into some of the deepest human feelings. Feelings about sacred places, tribal kinship, hierarchical status, and the responsibilities of a continuous lineage…non-clinical managers rarely understand the *volksgeist*, the cultural pride of the clinical teams involved, a feeling that may have built up over many years.[98]

More than 20 years after the event, the initial turmoil and disarray of the early years of the merger have been largely absorbed into a broader, positive narrative about the long-term benefits for both institutions. Nevertheless, the powerful and emotional responses of interviewees to remembering that period of flux reflects the depth and strength of the connection between professional identities and the specific institution.

Guy's Phase III building

At the outset of the merger, Guy's staff believed their superior facilities would give them the edge and that the 'state of the art' Philip Harris House would be a prime asset.

> We had a big surgical wing which was only about 20 years
> old. We had a tower which was 32 storeys high which
> was brand new. We had a brand-new building (Philip
> Harris House) which was frozen in time with the merger,
> but nevertheless was state of the art and is functioning
> beautifully now. But we were told that our facilities were
> of inferior building quality to those at St Thomas'. [99]

Guy's Phase III building was part of the post-war rebuilding
programme. The original intention had been for Phase III to follow
on after the completion of the Tower in the 1970s. In the event the
project did not advance until the Lewisham and North Southwark
District Health Authority's strategic review in 1984. This set out plans
for developing acute healthcare provision within the district on two
sites: Guy's to the north and Lewisham Hospital to the south. The
development was approved in principle by the Treasury in December
1986 with costs estimated at £35.5 million, and the Department of
Health promoted Phase III as 'a model of cooperation' between
the public and private sectors. Guy's implementation of clinical
directorates was a positive influence on the decision. Forty-five per
cent of the original funding was contributed by the Special Trustees
and private and charitable donors and included a £5m donation from
Philip Harris in recognition of which the building was to be named
'Philip Harris House'. [100] Work began in July 1990 and the occasion was
marked by a brochure which included a message of congratulations
from Kenneth Clarke as Secretary of State for Health. Completion
was scheduled for 1994 and it was, remarked Sandra Carnall Ferrelly
who worked on the initial development, the embodiment of a dream
which would realise the creation of 'the best in hospital facilities this
country has to offer'.

> The seeds of becoming a Trust were very much in the
> design of Philip Harris House, and we looked at how to
> design a new hospital for the twenty-first century, how

could we do things differently from the traditional ways? We came up with this view that if the ward and the out-patient department and the offices of a particular speciality were co-located you didn't have people walking between different places. Some of the doctors had three offices. Total waste of space. We said no, there are standard sizes…very much of the Trust emergence was tied in the new building. How can we do things differently? How can we do things better and cheaper? [101]

But the future of Philip Harris House was thrown into jeopardy by the announcement in February 1994 that the A&E alongside other acute services would be sited at St Thomas'. Investors revolted against the plans. The Philip and Pauline Harris Charitable Trust had promised to contribute £5 million and began proceedings to recover the initial £2 million donated.[102] The Imperial Cancer Research Fund had invested £1.7 million to enable the development of a comprehensive hub of research and treatment for breast cancer. Professor Nicholas Wright, Director of Clinical Research, asked for assurances that if the services were to move to the St Thomas' site, they would be assured the same quality of accommodation: 'otherwise there is no question whatsoever that we should have to demand our money back'.[103] The original plan was for the building to house a range of out-patient, day-care, and elective in-patient surgical services alongside research and teaching facilities. But the changes meant that only 75 per cent of the space was able to be used as originally intended. The remainder of space was to be remodified for a Planned Care Centre.

Alongside the disputes about the use of the building, the wildly escalating costs of Phase III led to an investigation by the National Audit Office in 1998 into the overrunning of costs and delays on the building. One of the contributory factors had been the insistence by the RHA that each of the four disciplines involved in the building programme – architecture, mechanical and electrical engineering, structural engineering, and quantity surveying – had to be put to competitive tender. To create a strong team Guy's had wanted to invite composite quotes so that bidders could put together their own teams. Instead, they were overruled, and it became increasingly difficult to maintain strong relations. The matter was finally settled through litigation.[104]

Boosting morale

As the merger arrangements across services and teams slowly bedded down, a new sense of community began to emerge. This was epitomised by the introduction of an annual staff pantomime in 1995 which continued until 2009. Led by Betsy Morley, senior site nursing manager at Guy's who continued the role in the new Trust, and Guy's hospital chaplain, Neville Smith, the initiative began as a way of trying to boost staff morale 'because it was so bad'. Betsy and her friends from the Nurses' League were discussing how awful things were at Guy's, 'it felt almost as though it was the end of everything' and they came up with the idea of a pantomime as a way of bringing people together. Not surprisingly, the immediate figure who came to mind was the Secretary of State, Virginia Bottomley.

> Virginia Bottomley, poor woman, came in for all the stick because we hated Virginia Bottomley. I said, we could do *Red Riding Hood* or *Who's Afraid of Virginia Wolf*, and we'll make the wolf Virginia Bottomley. We thought this was hysterical. I said, first of all we've got to find the pantomime script. Well, it's not easy to find a pantomime anywhere. Most of them were very crude to be honest and not, to my mind, suitable. So, I said, well I should think we could write it, we know the story, don't we? And it gave me the opportunity to be completely, non-politically correct in every possible aspect, having a go at this poor woman in Parliament and all the rest of it.[105]

Both institutions had well-established theatrical traditions. St Thomas' had Christmas shows which took the form of pantomimes or sketches with music. Instant Sunshine, which continues to the present and became an internationally renowned musical group, began when Peter Christie, Alan Maryon Davies and David Barlow came together to perform at the Christmas show.

> Peter had a string of these original songs, originally written for the St Thomas' Christmas show and it was on the strength of those songs that we formed the little group, Instant Sunshine. We just did a few parties, 21sts and bar mitzvahs and eventually we got hired by a restaurant in Mayfair and we used to sing there every Friday night for 17 years.[106]

Guy's productions were well-known for their strong use of satire to make humorous, political points about Guy's Hospital. The Greenwood Theatre which was opened on the Guy's site in 1975 was used to stage the productions.

> Sir Rowan Boland started theatrical productions after the war, and he was very good, he wrote many of them. They were brilliant. I've still got some of the music from them. And they turned out people who went far, like Tony Bron, who was Eleanor Bron's brother. They'd always have a theme of what was going on at the hospital at the time, whatever it was, scurrilous as it may be. But Betsy said, I'm not doing that, we'll do a panto, we'll do a traditional, good old-fashioned panto, because we'd got the Greenwood Theatre, which had been a bit of an Irishman's gift in the first instance. But we could invite the local population in. So, it was done with children in mind...they loved seeing people making a fool of themselves and the mistakes. But it was more professional than one would think, but it was

still very amateur. It was difficult enough getting rehearsals with people on shift and all the rest of it, so quite often you were rehearsing with a wall.[107]

The first performance was put on with very little scenery and only a few costumes, but the theatre was packed with people. Betsy and her friends had envisaged it would be a one-off event, but it was introduced by the theatre manager as the Guy's and St Thomas' Annual Pantomime. That led to a 14-year run of pantomime performances that involved people from all parts of the new Trust, including the Chief Executive, Tim Matthews.

> We started the pantomime. It was a way of getting people together from both Guy's and St Thomas', the two hospitals, from all levels of staff...I mean for three years Tim Matthews took the role of Dame. Now, that was such a boost for the staff because there were porters in it, there was everybody in it. I used to write and direct it, and it was always my little joke after the auditions. I would line people up and I can remember Tim standing there with all these others looking a bit uncomfortable – some of them because he was standing there – and I said, this is the Trust pantomime, and as such you'll meet people you've never seen before or heard of, and this is one of the big advantages of the pantomime. We all have a great time, and we'd get to know people. I said, there is one thing. Nobody is more important than the next person, whatever their job in the Trust. There is only one person who is more important, and that is me as Director. And this went down well. Well, I hope it did. They all came back for more.[108]

The pantomime also featured cameo appearances by Simon Hughes, MP for Bermondsey. In 2006 when Charles Kennedy, leader of the Liberal Democrats, resigned unexpectedly, Simon as President had to abandon his role of the Sultan in Alibaba and the Almost Forty Thieves. In 2009 the decision was taken to end the pantomime series in light of 'rumours' that a new cancer centre was to replace the Greenwood Theatre.[109] Bringing staff across the merged organisations together in this way had proved highly effective in developing new friendships and networks across the merged organisation.

Moving forwards

At the outset of the merger, the Trust Board agreed on a set of measures to encourage staff to transition to a single Trust. Everybody's title and role were Trust-wide, and staff would only be given a site-based title for operational reasons. Success was to be recognised when staff began to speak about a single institution.

> When we heard people start talking about Guy's and St Thomas' more often than they started talking about Guy's *or* St Thomas' then that would be a real signal of how things were.[110]

Staff who were too distraught and saddened by the merger to continue in their posts chose to leave. Betsy Morley, chair of the Nurse's League, remembers how animosity ran deep: 'the only people who never accepted it of course, were the old guard from the Guy's Hospital Nurses' League, who could never come to terms with it. Never did come to terms with it at all. And when we had our final fling in 2010, which was just the most wonderful day, they still were feeling that we'd had Guy's stolen from us'.[111] But most staff remained and the natural turnover in junior medical staff, nursing, paramedics, and ancillary staff helped bring in new generations who only knew Guy's and St Thomas' as a merged Trust. Sandra Carnell Ferrelly reflected that it tended to be younger people from St Thomas' who participated in the pantomime and did not harbour the memory of the merger.[112]

You come straight into a place, you don't know that Guy's and St Thomas' haven't always been Guy's and St Thomas'. So, the pantomime did help in putting behind some of the issues. And Tim Matthews, the chief executive, he played the dame a couple of times, and he was a nice enough guy.

After a horrendously busy few years, Tim Matthews describes the period around 1996/97 as a point when things were settling down.

I think a lot of things really came together in about '96, '97, with the approval of the business plan. We started to change some things, we had an agreed plan for both the contractual completion and then the refitting of the new building at Guy's, at the same time, the medical schools were moving into being part of King's College and had developed a complementary plan which we helped to finance to develop services at Guy's. So, you know, the job was never finished, but it felt like, you know, once we got to '96, '97 with the business plan approved, with the cardiac department coming together, with the maternity services plan to come together, with the new building at Guy's opening and with the agreement to close and move the emergency services to St Thomas' that, you know, if we hadn't broken the back of the problems, we'd got beyond the point of no return. And people were beginning to talk about the Trust as Guy's *and* Thomas' rather than, you know, this is Guy's and this is Thomas'. There was a huge amount still to do, but I think one of the lessons from that is for organisations like this, you know, there are some things you can do quickly to some extent, you can set the rules and set the agenda, but actually these things take, you know, take a huge amount of time to work their way through and, you know, I suspect continue to do so.[113]

Through the swirl of merger activities, wider shifts to make health services more responsive to patient needs were taking place. Since the 1980s, patient organisations had lobbied for rights and transparency – such as access to medical records – and the notion of the patient as consumer emerged with the new business-like culture of accountability.[114] In July 1991, the Citizen's Charter was introduced across public and private sector services. This set out organisational standards and methods for measuring performance, and Brian Edwards, regional general manager of the Trent Regional Health Authority, translated this into the NHS Patient's Charter although patient groups deemed the Charter to be a disappointment and expressed concern that it would not address collective aims such as improving inequalities within the NHS.[115] The New Labour Government, led by Tony Blair, came to power in 1997, and introduced a raft of policy initiatives with the overarching aim of reducing waiting lists and improving services. Health organisations were put under increasing pressure to report data to assess performance. In 1999 it came to light at Guy's and St Thomas' that patients in plastic surgery and orthopaedics were being suspended from waiting lists to avoid reporting breaches of the 18-month maximum wait. An internal investigation found that there was 'a belief' by junior staff that it was in the Trust's interest to suspend patients rather than suffer breaches and that this practice was supported by senior management. The Trust Board concluded that the matter was one of 'corporate responsibility' and no individuals should be singled out for disciplinary action.[116] Rivett notes that the pressure to hit targets meant that it was not uncommon for hospitals to manipulate information in some cases.[117]

Guy's and St Thomas' had been aware of the need to make patients the focus of how care was planned and delivered before the merger. Karen Caines explained in Chapter 4 how the new Guy's and Lewisham Trust had begun to innovate the delivery of maternity services to benefit patients by having local ante-natal clinics to save women having to travel into London. Tim Matthews described the shift as a 'broader, cultural movement in public service and health services'.

> It was never a criticism, implicit or otherwise, of the quality of care that individual clinicians or clinical teams gave to individual patients, but it was things like how we organised clinics, you know, as much for the convenience of patients as for the attendance of doctors, that's one example. How we responded to complaints. We took complaints seriously, how we set up and investigated where we had risks or accidents and that we learnt from those and that the way we informed, you know, and greeted and welcomed patients, you know, increasingly felt like, you know, something that was not a retail experience, but, you know, they felt much more like a consumer of service than a victim of professional judgement. There isn't one answer to that, that's a whole array of things, you know, some of which were changing anyway, but I think I and my team had a very strong sense that, you know, that was the service we wanted.[118]

Addressing and meeting patients' needs went well beyond the better organisation of service delivery. One poignant example was the introduction in the 1990s of an annual service for parents who had suffered miscarriages, stillbirths and/or abortions. An awareness of the need for these tragedies to be recognised and acknowledged had begun in the mid-1980s. Michael Cooley, Guy's Roman Catholic chaplain, remembers a terrible scene with a mother who had a stillbirth and wanted him to say prayers and talk with her: 'the midwife was so offhand because it wasn't the done thing at that time. Stillbirth was just disposed of'. That led to a discussion about what needed to change, and some study days were held in the maternity unit to discuss bereavement and help midwives cope better with the needs of patients. On one occasion, a mother refused to have a caesarean section for religious reasons, even though she had been visited and reassured by a minister that it would be all right. 'The midwives had to stand round and watch the baby die.' The midwives asked Michael how they could make sense of such an event: 'in the Western world we would say a caesarean is the will of God. It's a wonderful discovery and a gift of God. But if you've got no contact with that sort of hospital or facility you have to take it within your culture'.[119] In the early 1990s, chaplain Neville Smith began an annual service for lost babies in response to the grief he witnessed in maternity services at Guy's. He recollects, 'There was a need for some kind of service, some kind of ritual, some kind of prayers, some kind of observance to say that this was a real person. This person had actually existed, and we can grieve for this baby or because of this baby who didn't actually make it.' This included commemorating miscarriages, still births and abortions. Word began to get around that Guy's had introduced this support for bereaved parents.

> One of the saddest things that ever happened to me was because of this. This mother came along. She'd lost two children early on. Miscarriages. The only trace that she had were two appointment cards for the antenatal clinic, and she brought these two cards along and, I don't know, I devised some little ritual, service to mark these two lives that had never come to anything, and we lit a couple of candles. But this had happened a good number of years, 10, 15 years ago, but she was still within herself grieving for these two early miscarriages. She'd had these two children that she'd never actually brought to term.[120]

The response of the chaplaincy to patient needs is one example of how the historical cultures of Guy's and St Thomas' as remote, autonomous institutions were beginning to shift. Following the merger, local GPs were critical of the way in which the Trust operated, and they became 'powerful allies' in encouraging the Trust to 'get real and be more engaged'.

> The work was increasingly being, sort of, prompted and supported by things like waiting lists and waiting time initiatives which were, you know, in effect, saying to hospitals and clinicians, you've got to change your priorities and time and access is as important for people and society, at large, as your individual judgement as to whether Mr X or Mrs Y needs to be seen next. So that was, like, one of the big cultural changes going on; the other which was much more around the strategy was trying to build across clinical teams, this sense of how we're going to create bigger, better departments, how we're going to use that to, you know, create something that's more than just some of the parts, whether that's in terms of clinical care, teaching or research.[121]

The need to create a more open, inclusive culture around public and patient involvement with health services led to Frank Dobson, Secretary of State for Health, introducing new rules around appointments for non-executive roles in NHS Trusts. Patricia Moberly had lived in the area since the 1960s and served on Lambeth Council and the North Lewisham and Southwark DHA. She was also a schoolteacher and as recounted in Chapter 4, 'I'd get very, very irritated in how difficult it was for people to get jobs here, particularly here in St Thomas'. Previously, non-executive roles had been filled by 'tapping people on the shoulder' but they were now advertised for the first time: 'They wanted more of a mix. They only had one woman at the time, and I think they wanted more women. They wanted more local people. They wanted a wider spectrum of interests.'[122] Patricia joined the Guy's and St Thomas' Board in 1997. She retired from teaching in 1998 and had a cancer operation at St

Thomas'. The then chairman, Kenneth Eaton, was asked to stay on as no replacement had been found and Patricia decided to apply: 'rather to my surprise, I got it'. None of the previous chairmen had connections to Lambeth: 'they were all good people in their way, but they were political appointees. My predecessor was an Admiral of the Fleet and lived in Hampshire, and his main claim to fame was that he'd been responsible for Trident. He was a very good person, but he had no connection with this hospital or with the local area'.[123] Patricia took up her appointment in 1999. Tim Matthews retired as Chief Executive in 2000 and Jonathan Michael became the new Chief Executive. Chapter 6 will show how Patricia was to have enormous influence on reshaping the merged Trust in the 2000s addressing many of the historical hidden influences including freemasonry.

Conclusion

In March 1998, as the tumultuous decade began to draw to a close, Her Majesty Queen Elizabeth II visited to formally open Thomas Guy House – the final name for the building originally intended to be named Philip Harris House. The opening marked 'a new era in healthcare at Guy's and St Thomas', proclaimed the official brochure.[124] The building exemplified the highest specifications of hospital building including an integrated 'computer-based control system encompassing all of the engineering, plant and services in relation to the internal environment of the building', noted Graham Perry, Project Director. It signified the completion of the Guy's rebuilding programme planned in 1946. A senior group of clinicians had sketched out their vision for the building in the early 1980s. They imagined the new building as a space for clinical innovation, involving the delivery of system-based care to patients through departments that brought together the range of specialists needed to treat specific conditions. It is unlikely that they could have anticipated then, a scenario in which the completed building would be part of the merged Guy's and St Thomas' Trust estate. Nor indeed did those present at the opening, despite knowing that the merger between UMDS and King's College London was about to complete, have any inkling that in a decade's time, they would be part of the first cohort of academic health science centres.

CHAPTER SIX

Beyond Hospital Walls, 1990-1999

Overview

A longside the merger of Guy's and St Thomas' NHS Trusts there was also the merger of UMDS with King's College London, which established the merged medical and dental schools as part of a multi-faculty institution. Taking place in parallel to the merger of the Guy's and St Thomas' Trusts, the merger between UMDS and King's College took around eight years to complete with myriad logistical and regulatory obstacles needing to be overcome alongside the day-to-day challenges of managing merged student cohorts and curriculum change. It marked the end point of a debate begun in 1968 when the Royal Commission on Medical Education, led by Lord Todd, had recommended that medical and dental students should undertake their non-clinical training in a multi-faculty environment rather than a free-standing medical school. The joining of the hospital Trusts also led to the creation of the Guy's and St Thomas' Charity which brought together the hospitals' endowment funds and established new criteria to make the Charity more fit for purpose.

Rationalising London medical education

In 1990 London still had 12 standalone medical schools despite recommendations dating from the 1968 Royal Commission that the overall number should be reduced, and stand-alone medical schools should move to becoming part of multi-faculty institutions. The need for change was becoming ever more pressing. Science had developed significantly during the 1980s aided by the advances in biotechnology. The medical schools' pre-clinical departments were responding to this expansion in sciences by introducing new specialties into teaching, for example, immunology. But establishing immunology departments in each medical school was costly and led to the duplication of facilities across sites. Furthermore, the argument that integrating medical schools into multi-faculty institutions would extend opportunities across education and research, enabling research to span from science research at the bench, to clinical research at the bedside, had gained momentum after the introduction of the Research Assessment Exercise (RAE) in 1986. The RAE evaluated the quality of research in higher education institutions and was linked to financial allocations, which meant no medical school could ignore the consequences of not performing well in research activities.[1] Another concern was that as standalone institutions, medical schools would be vulnerable to the risk of medical training transferring to the NHS.

> The NHS was always predatory about training doctors and nurses, and so on. And we all felt that the training they would get at the hands of the NHS would be merciless as regards the finances that would be put into education. In the end, the NHS is in this terrible position that, when the finances squeeze, it must go to patient services, and research and education get all the cuts. So, in many ways, it would be better to go into the university system and to try and maintain it, which is going back to the Flexner Report in America.[2]

Thus, the pressures and drivers in the wider context created an acceptance across London, albeit reluctant, that further medical school mergers were inevitable. 'The writing was on the wall,' was a phrase several interviewees used when reflecting on this time. UMDS took the view that it was better to find their own solution to the problem, rather than wait for one enforced by the Government. An initial meeting was held in private on Christmas Eve 1986 between Ian Cameron, Principal of UMDS, Tim Clark, Dean of UMDS, and Stewart Sutherland, Principal of King's College London. The day was chosen particularly to minimise the risk of anyone noticing Stewart Sutherland's visit to Guy's. The meeting was positive although it was acknowledged that a merger 'would be a hard path'. There was no immediate action but in autumn 1990 John Beynon replaced Sutherland as Principal of King's College and Ian Cameron went to meet him.

> He seemed alright, and King's seemed the sort of institution we could do business with. The talks started. There were talks and talks and talks between John Beynon and myself. I talk a lot, but he talked more. We had little dinners in little restaurants where we thought no one would see us all the way round Westminster. I remember my wife saying, there better had be a John Beynon. By Christmas 1990 I wrote a paper in which I outlined all the options that UMDS might have, and these were in order to answer the questions around larger departments, more basic sciences, multi-faculty links and so on. It didn't seem right that students should go straight from school into a medical and dental ghetto and then come out as qualified doctors and dentists without ever meeting anyone who did anything else. That seemed wrong educationally. And looking around, well the obvious solution was to join with King's academic departments.[3]

The discussion progressed through a series of working parties and dinners, spurred on by the expectation that the Tomlinson report (commissioned in 1991) would make recommendations on mergers.

When Ian Cameron returned from holiday in the summer of 1992, expecting to sign the agreement with John Beynon, he found that Arthur Lucas had replaced Beynon as Acting Principal at King's. Fortunately, this change in leadership did not disrupt the process and the agreement was signed. The next six or so years were dominated by merger processes and after the successful passing of the King's College Merger Bill in 1997, the formal merger took place on 1 August 1998. This created three new schools: the Guy's, King's, and St Thomas' Schools of Medicine, of Dentistry and of Biomedical Sciences, and reconfigured part of the former King's College School of Life, Basic Medical & Health Sciences as the new School of Health & Life Sciences.

Siting the new schools

Just as with the merger of Guy's and St Thomas' Trusts, discussions on how the UMDS and King's merger would be effected across the various sites was fraught with difficulties and obstacles. The original aspiration was for 'a strong UMDS on St Thomas' and full use of the splendid new facilities at Guy's'.[4] But Virginia Bottomley's decision to concentrate acute and specialist services at St Thomas' created a natural push towards developing Guy's as a centre for teaching and research alongside some health services. The appraisal of the case for co-locating UMDS and King's, solely on the Guy's site, proved to be 'neither feasible in economic terms nor affordable'.[5] Eventually a scheme was agreed that involved merger across three sites whereby life, basic medical and health sciences would be consolidated on the Guy's site; health sciences would be consolidated at Cornwall House; and all other KCL departments would remain on the Strand.[6]

The merger process proved to be hugely challenging with logistical and regulatory obstacles dogging progress, as well as the difficulties of managing the sheer number of students. After the 1980s' mergers, the pre-clinical cohort was 195 students at UMDS and 105 students at King's.[7] By 1998 the combined medical school had an intake of 343 students, the highest in the UK.[8] This increased to 401 students in 2001 with a further increase of 50 students in 2002 through the Extended Medical Programme.[9] The UMDS merger had proved tricky enough in terms of merging teaching schools with different cultures and histories, and the King's merger was complicated by the fact that UMDS was merging with a university.[10] Arthur Lucas did not doubt that the merger was going to take a long period of time to become fully effective.

> I never believed it would fully function until at least ten years after the formal merger, that's partly because you've got five- or six-years' cohorts of students completing the courses which they'd started. You've got, particularly in London hospital medical schools, enormously strong, *enormously strong*, commitment to the hospital in which you trained, because most of the people teaching at Thomas' trained at Thomas', most of the people teaching at Barts trained at Barts, and so on, and so on. And until they began to be diluted out by newer staff you wouldn't really get that sort of cultural integration.[11]

Untangling the ownership of properties so that the physical infrastructure to support the merger could be developed, for example, was a hugely complicated task, and Arthur Lucas, Cyril Chantler, Dean of UMDS and Tim Matthews, Chief Executive of Guy's and St Thomas', decided to refer the matter to William Wells, chairman of the South Thames NHS Executive who was also knowledgeable about property. Various deals were done, including a 'single vote transfer' between health and education so that some of the property owned by the NHS was transferred to King's, some for redevelopment and some leased back to the Trust. The arrangements did not totally satisfy either side, noted Arthur Lucas, but they were accepted as 'eminently fair'.

These transfers were necessary to make the site viable to occupy for the academic functions of the merged College, especially the science departments...The 'single vote transfer' was as far as I now understand it, a book-keeping exercise by central Government, transferring the property en bloc to KCL, adding it to the 'Treasury interest' in KCL property (ie a set of restrictions that apply to the disposal of such property that would need approval by the Government). From the KCL point of view we had to forgo actual rent on the property that Guy's-St Thomas' Hospitals continued to occupy, and there were rules about when the tenants could be evicted and so on. We also had to take on the responsibility of buildings that turned out to be in extremely poor repair that cost a great deal to bring into use. But it cleared the obstacles. So, Sir William Wells was a key player in unblocking the log jam.[12]

The financial arrangements were complicated, and the leadership was forced to think innovatively about the options for financing the merger and managing the risks of the operation. Knowing that Guy's Phase III building had vastly overrun the estimated budget and timelines for completion left no room for complacency about these issues.

King's was able to bring the sale of properties to the party, UMDS was able to bring cash to the party and, of course, once we went down what was described as, and what started off as, an early form of PFI financing, that won the brownie points with the Government at the time. I say it like that because it turned out not to be the model that government had been pushing. Essentially what the College did was to say we'll sell these properties at Kensington and Chelsea, and we need to refurbish and build other properties. To avoid the risk of these things getting out of kilter – the buildings not being ready at the right time – we invited a consortium to do the work so that part of the trick was that they would not get vacant possession of the potential residential properties at Chelsea and Kensington, until they'd finished the work on the academic functions. So that was a major risk reduction from the point of view of the College. It did not need to have the component that has been bedevilling a lot of the NHS PFIs and that is the transfer of ownership of the asset. We never transferred ownership of any asset, other than the ones we were actually selling. We transferred risk and that worked well.[13]

Under the terms of the merger, the rights, properties, and liabilities of UMDS assets would be transferred to King's College. To allay fears that King's College may be tempted to sell some of the assets they acquired, a body known as the Continuing Trustees of UMDS was set up for a period of ten years. It safeguarded the risk of properties or land being sold off as any change in use other than those associated with student education and research required the support of the Trustees.

The sale of any asset that was owned by the UMDS at the date of merger could not be undertaken by King's College unless those trustees agreed. So, it was prevention against the accusation of asset stripping. The major concern was sports grounds, people were very dedicated to their sports grounds, and of course, it was seen that a lot of these sports grounds are situated in highly-desirable residential areas, and so there was a fear that they would be stripped. So, there was a great list of properties in an annex to the Act. I don't know who thought of that, but it was quite a clever solution.[14]

The merger had to be ratified by Parliament and the most straightforward and least contentious option appeared to be through a Private Member's Bill, and Peter Brooke, MP for the Cities of London and Westminster, agreed to take this on. But readings of the Bill took place in the run-up to the 1997 General Election, and Simon Hughes MP for Bermondsey and Southwark who was a vociferous supporter of Guy's made numerous objections which delayed the process significantly.[15] 'It was awful. It was absolutely awful. We were running out of time. We couldn't sign our contracts for sale of property, we couldn't sign anything else till we had the Merger Bill,' remembered Arthur Lucas.

> I mean [Simon] was quite blunt about it, he said to us, you know, you'll get it through in the end, you'll get it through in the end, no I'm not going to stop it forever. He took Cyril and I out on to the terrace after one of these things where it was supposed to have been debated and he objected and so it was just passed over. He said it'll come, it'll come, don't worry about it, it'll come. But it was just one of those awkwardnesses; it was because it was a very political time with that important election.

Eventually in 1997 the Bill went through the House of Commons followed by the House of Lords.

Bedding down

All London medical and dental schools were aware of the changing environment and the broad shifts to integrating schools within multi-faculty institutions. Amongst UMDS and King's staff, attitudes towards the merger had been reasonably positive, although at UMDS there was sadness that the merger with King's would break the historical traditions of close relationships between the hospitals and medical schools that had been maintained through the UMDS merger. King's medical school had become part of King's College London in 1983 and was already embedded in the wider institutional structures and processes of the university. But for UMDS, the prospect of the schools sitting within governance and leadership structures that did not necessarily align to the core purposes and ambitions of the medical and dental schools was concerning. Inevitably, both sides expressed fears that the merger could prove to be a takeover. UMDS was a larger medical school than King's; King's was part of a university institution.

> At UMDS there was a distinct feeling that the administrative arrangements of the larger institution would prevail and that there was little question of taking the best of each and it was several years before some of these innovations introduced at UMDS reappeared within King's College London.[16]

But even though King's medical school was part of the university it was based in Camberwell and in practice operated almost like 'a satellite medical school' and did not take much account for example of the wider King's regulations.[17] From the King's perspective the merger threatened to disrupt the geographical independence that the senior leadership had established.[18]

The leadership team made efforts to address these fears by establishing a lead-in period as Arthur Lucas explained.

> I think that the most important point is that the establishing of trust between people in mergers is quite critically important. I won't go into the details of how that was done but I think we used a very sensitive procedure, including shadowing and all sorts of things, for example cross-representation on councils, so I was a member of the

UMDS council for the last two years of its existence, and vice versa. So those things were done.

Adrian Eddleston, Dean of King's School of Medicine and Dentistry, and Gwyn Williams, Dean of UMDS, came to 'a gentleman's agreement' about their role. Adrian became Dean of the merged school for two years until his retirement in 2000; then Gwyn became Dean until 2004. Adrian was very positive about the merger benefits.

When I was asked to become the first dean of the merged medical schools of Guy's, King's and St Thomas', I'd already had experience of working in a multi-faculty university. I was Guy's trained originally, so I could see both sides of the equation, and I was also able to be enthusiastic about what King's would bring to the equation, what the University would bring to the equation, because working with multi-faculty colleagues, not just science colleagues, but the whole plethora of the multi-faculties in the University was most rewarding to me. It reminded me of my Oxford days, which is where I started off, and it brought back the vigour of listening to the intellectual debate. One of the important departments that helped us with our revamped curriculum and the whole of the entry of access students into medicine, for example, was the education department of King's. Here was a chance to benefit from others' thinking in a quite different way than one would in a stand-alone medical school. So, I thought that was brilliant and I was able to bring that experience to the merger.

Nevertheless, bringing the departments together of the merged schools proved trickier than Adrian had anticipated.

How amazed I was to find that UMDS was not the *United* Medical and Dental Schools at all. When I came to become

Dean of the merged schools the first thing I did was to try and work out who should be heads of department and deputy heads of department, heads of research groupings, et cetera. I went along to St Thomas' on one occasion and said, could you tell me, who is the head of diabetes for UMDS? and they said, do you mean the head of St Thomas' diabetes? So you can imagine the tussle of trying to decide how to form the departments to get that balance exactly right, and that's another story and was a major task to accomplish.[19]

Adrian recounted this story at the Witness Seminar and Ian Cameron who had instigated merger discussions interjected, 'Diabetes, as you know very well, that was an impossibility to bring together. Getting [the consultants] to agree to anything was beyond anyone. God knows I tried!'[20] But not all areas proceeded so smoothly as establishing the leadership roles.

Before the merger concerns had been raised that UMDS' assets were 'comfortably in the black whereas King's was in the red', though as Arthur noted earlier, King's brought properties as assets. Stephen Challacombe was on the UMDS' Finance Committee and remembers, 'wading through late at night, hundreds of pages of figures to see whether we'd missed anything – it was quite daunting'.[21] UMDS' strong financial status had come about through a radical reorganisation of budgets across the various medical divisions during the first half of the 1990s. Principal, Cyril Chantler, and David Potter, Chairman of the Finance Committee, gave divisions their own budgets and then encouraged them to collaborate to get better value by sharing resources.

We had probably one of the strongest balance sheets of any medical school in the country; we had 20 million quid in the bank, we were a really solid institution. We made a profit but called it a fund for reinvestment. It seemed quite radical at the time but was pretty successful.[22]

So initially it was a shock for an institution, accustomed to having excellent long-term and everyday financial control, to lose this through the merger.

The first negative effect I'll mention was not evident until after merger, and as far as I know, and I could not find any evidence of it when I tried to find out, there was no what I would call a prenuptial agreement of the finances. To put it in a nutshell, the UMDS funds that we were used to using disappeared overnight, and they were all now part of King's College funding and there were no facilities for doing the sort of things that one had with access to various funds because the UMDS no longer existed, therefore the funds didn't exist, they had disappeared into King's College. I'm not in favour of deans having a large slice of finances allotted to them, but they do need some to act as oil to keep the wheels turning and that was a very difficult time.[23]

The overnight disappearance of funds had immediate and enormous consequences for the everyday experiences of students and staff. For example, the funds allocated to support UMDS student societies were no longer available and although the intention was that UMDS students could join the King's Music Society, the King's Mountaineering Society, and so on, UMDS societies had been hubs that attracted members from the hospitals including nurses and ancillary staff in varying degrees. As discussed previously in relation to the UMDS merger, sports became a flashpoint for the strong associations between identities and institution.

The longest running arguments and points of high feeling were the Rowing Club and the Rugby Team, partly related to the fact that the Guy's Hospital Rugby Club is not known to many people but is the oldest rugby club in the United Kingdom. And the fact that it would possibly lose its name under the merger caused a lot of anger, and not only from the current rugby players, but from all the past ones as well.[24]

After the merger David Potter was promoted as the Treasurer to King's College as a whole and found it tricky to get people to see the merger from a business perspective.

The whole point of a merger is you put something together and you find the best person to do that job. You don't slot people in because you won't achieve any benefit out of it. I know it's not a business, but it's got to be business-like.[25]

At senior level, many of the immediate difficulties were caused by a fundamental lack of understanding at King's senior leadership level about the intricacies of medical and dental school training programmes. In medicine, the General Medical Council (GMC) sets out what students are required to learn to become doctors. For senior staff in UMDS it was second nature to look over their shoulder at two masters. But staff at King's found it difficult to engage with the concept that an outside body would decide the curriculum for a faculty in King's College. In practical terms the demands of UMDS curricula meant that students did not operate within traditional university terms. The pressure from King's was to 'squash the medical school three years' curriculum into a more conventional university type year but still it did not work and that was a very time-consuming exercise'.

I found myself over the years trying to teach the philosophy of being part of a thriving young university to my clinical colleagues, and trying to get King's College London to understand what it means to have a clinical component when all the regulations that they'd been used to had nothing to do with clinical students.[26]

The logistical challenges of merging medical, dental, and biomedical teaching were daunting. For example in the early period there were five different curricula in operation which complicated the processes of external validation by the GMC and Higher Education funding bodies, reflected Hywel Thomas: 'it was a nightmare doing the teaching quality exercise, because we had to really explain to the people coming to visit us, now, you're going to judge us against five different curricula'. He noted how the merger challenges were intensified by the wider context of the RAE which meant that the medical school's income was directly affected by the quality of the research.

> The worst thing really was the fact that you could never reach a status quo. You thought you'd reached a plateau and then there was another cliff to climb and, of course, at the same time, the Government required all members of teaching staff to be research-active at the school. So that put pressure on you to publish as much as you can and get as much research as you could, because the income of the school depended very much on the research quality exercise. A change of half a grade, or something, meant you'd lost millions, so there was a lot of pressure on individual members of staff dealing with curricular changes, dealing with research pressures, grants became tighter and more difficult to obtain and students got more demanding in a way. Previously they would be very happy with the lectures, then, of course, they wanted handouts and they wanted all kinds of things, so students got more and more demanding, quite naturally, because, you know, they were expecting a lot more from their teachers, having

experienced changes in the school. So individual members of staff very, very often were under tremendous pressure.[27]

The arrangements around clinical teaching and the intersections between the medical school and the NHS were also a source of tension. Most clinical teaching happened in the hospitals and was delivered by hospital consultants and the more senior junior staff.

> Of course, these people are not employed by the University and a lot of our students went out to peripheral hospitals, down in Brighton for example or in mid-Kent, and they would appoint a new consultant who would therefore have teaching responsibility. And several members at King's College were aghast at the fact that people were being appointed to teach students of King's College who had not been interviewed to be teachers at King's College.[28]

The historical symbiosis between the hospital and the medical school had led to medical school space being embedded within hospital space. For example, there were departments including laboratories and offices that belonged to the medical school but were housed within hospital space. These issues were eventually resolved through cooperation that entailed 'a lot of hard work'.[29]

This lack of recognition of the specific day-to-day operations of the medical school coloured this early period and required intensive input to resolve. This was despite the fact that King's College Medical School had been reincorporated into King's College in 1983. The King's merger, like the UMDS merger, had had no significant impact on day-to-day operations hence the underappreciation of the needs of a medical school compared to a university faculty. For example, King's College expected to have student residences occupied for the three university terms and to use them for income generation at other times of the year.

All the residences that were UMDS were now King's College, and students came to me one day distraught because they had received notices to quit their rooms at the end of the traditional university term so that they could be let out for conferences et cetera. Of course, they were still required to be in London studying the curriculum which does not follow the ordinary university terms. Now, you would have thought this could be solved with a quick telephone call. It turned into again a major, major problem which eventually had to be resolved, but really it was a very time consuming and, in my view, unnecessary discussion.[30]

Indeed, UMDS students were more resistant of the merger than UMDS staff who could appreciate the advantages more easily. Frank Ashley, previously Dean of the Dental School in UMDS, was appointed Dean of the Guy's, King's, and St Thomas' Dental Institute. Gwyn Williams, at that time Vice Dean of the merged medical school, shared a suite of offices with Frank and remembers him having a bruising encounter with the dental undergraduates.

He came back looking rather ashen from his confrontation with the students and he told me he had been berated as he had never been in his life by a female dental undergraduate who had stood up in the meeting. The essence of her anger was that she had never, ever applied to King's to do dentistry. She had applied to the UMDS Dental School. The merger was a complete betrayal of her trust et cetera, et cetera. I think he found it rather difficult to argue with this forceful young woman who was a mature student, had already done a degree and was obviously quite used to standing on her hind legs and arguing with top brass.[31]

As in previous mergers, the name of the new medical school was of utmost importance because it embedded the longer historical past.

When UMDS had formed in 1982 the students were vociferous about their dislike of losing their identity as either a Guy's or a St Thomas' student. But the merger had been gradually accepted and UMDS became a successful institution with a student body that was as proud and loyal to UMDS as previous generations had been to Guy's or St Thomas'. The merger with King's disrupted the equilibrium and the cycle started over again. Guy's, King's, and St Thomas' Schools of Medicine was rapidly abbreviated to GKT. Arthur Lucas resisted this forcefully.

> I was determined and I think most of my colleagues on the King's non-medical bits were determined to preserve the names of Thomas' and Guy's because they're very important historically, very important symbolically. Hence the way in which the epistructure of the medical schools came together as part of King's but as the Guy's, King's, and Thomas' Medical School, of King's College London technically, abbreviated to GKT inevitably of course. And I got into real trouble with students because I was insisting that they do not use GKT. They thought I was saying you've got to use King's, and I said, look no I wasn't, you've got to use the names Guy's and Thomas' otherwise there's no point in preserving them, if you just say GKT it means nothing to the outside world. So, I had interesting discussions with student unions, the medical bit, the members of the student unions about that. Once you pointed it out like most of them accepted it, and they're saying, he's not against using the names – he wants the full names used, but, of course, nobody does because it's so much easier just to say GKT.[32]

Whereas the merger between Guy's and St Thomas' medical and dental schools to form UMDS had been done on an amicable basis during the 1980s, the merger of UMDS with King's College London was much more adversarial. 'We talked about rivalry between Guy's and St Thomas', but that was nothing to the antipathy and animosity between UMDS and King's College.'[33] Ian reflected that some of his St Thomas' friends still think that it was 'one of the worst things that's ever happened. I keep quiet that it was me that signed the initial papers'.[34] Nevertheless, it was a smoother and more tolerable experience for staff than those involved in the merger of the nursing schools as Hywel Thomas reflects.

> So it was a challenging time, but I'm pleased to say that when UMDS finally signed all the merger documents, you know, we were a thriving institution, we were very cash rich, we didn't have much in the way of capital and when we signed, we handed over quite a lot of money to KCL, which, in retrospect, we should really have spent on setting up new chairs, et cetera, we had this cash there in reserve and so it was just signed and went into the King's coffers, I always regret that one aspect, but I think UMDS, for a short period, did very well and GKT actually got off the ground very, very quickly.[35]

The anticipated advantages of the merger were amply proven within a few years. The payoffs were increased research funding and high levels of recruitment. For example, the Dental Institute received the maximum rating in the 2001 Research Assessment Exercise. Students benefited from an enriched curriculum that offered Special Study Modules across a broad range of areas including the humanities. From a dean's perspective it was easy to attract excellent candidates for appointments because it was a large medical school within a multi-faculty institution which had a faculty of biomedical sciences.[36] Most importantly, though, it brought Guy's, St Thomas', and King's together and created the foundation for becoming an academic health science centre in the 2000s.

If I'd been a betting man in 1992, even when these talks were going on, and it had been said that the King's partners would be one of the first wave of academic medical partnerships, I'd have replied, you must be joking. So, I think a number of people in this room and outside, in getting through these mergers did an amazing job. And we ought to mention that sort of goodwill as it's a really positive story.[37]

Guy's and St Thomas' Charity

Guy's and St Thomas' Hospitals had benefited from endowment funds throughout their histories and with the establishment of the NHS in 1948, the funds were given charitable status. Apart from St Bartholomew's Hospital, Guy's and St Thomas' endowments were the largest in the UK with St Thomas' being the richer endowment. At St Thomas', new departments had often been enabled by endowment funding such as the acquisition of the first heart lung machine in 1958 and support for the renal transplant programme in 1969.[38] After the 1974 NHS reorganisation, the endowment funds were administered by the Special Trustees of each institution and had continued to provide a vital stream of funding across patient care and research. John Wyn Owen's view was that St Thomas' ability to be entrepreneurial, and create and shift the agenda, rested in large part on being able to access additional funding that was at a scale that would have been impossible from public funds.[39] Elaine Murphy who was appointed as professor of psychiatry at Guy's in 1983 described the Special Trustees as a 'slush fund' that was generous to new professors. The focus was solely on what was best for Guy's 'but not necessarily in the best interests of the NHS' and funding could often become a means of preventing enforced change from the district authorities.

For example, if there was a ward which should probably close, if they had enough clout through consultants or other people wanting to invest in it, they would invest money to support it to stay open. They could act incredibly autonomously and support things that they perceived were in the institution's best interest. You can't fault them for that, but it was sometimes not in the wider interests of the healthcare in the community.[40]

The Special Trustees were also able to bankroll the hospital in a financial crisis which 'prevented Guy's from going into the red many times. Those things protected the teaching hospitals from a lot of the NHS financial processes, so I thought they were a mixed blessing'.[41] Ian Gainsford was Dean of the Faculty of Clinical Dentistry at King's College London between 1983 and 1987. His view, as an outsider, was that access to these funds gave Guy's and St Thomas' 'a tremendous edge on the other hospitals in the RHA'. He remembers trying to raise £5m (a major part of the RHA budget for new developments) for a project for King's which was only at the first stage of planning when Guy's was at the building completion stage.

Guy's was able to attract all of the money available to the RHA because they could make a grant from their own funds of say £20 million and with that £5 million fund a project for £25 million which was more in the NHS' interest than to have a small project at King's.[42]

The Special Trustees also operated as a closed shop in the sense that Trustees were 'tapped on the shoulder' and told they were to be appointed and even when the appointments were formalised through the Department of Health, the names of potential Trustees were forwarded by others.

After the Guy's and St Thomas' Trust had been created, the Department of Health took the decision to appoint the same Special Trustees for the two hospitals in 1996, but this caused a great deal of unhappiness and Peter Lumsden who had chaired St Thomas' Special Trustees resigned in protest against the forced merger.[43] Tim Chessells had chaired the London Implementation Group (LIG) as part of the Tomlinson reforms and once that was disbanded he moved to chair the Legal Aid Board. He was approached by the Department of Health to ask if he would become one of the new Special Trustees and went on to become chair and lead the process of merging the Special Trustees. Geoffrey Shepherd was working as an NHS chief executive when he spotted an advertisement for the post of chief executive to the Special Trustees of the two hospitals. It attracted him because it was a job in which he could 'use money in quite creative ways and more creatively than if I'd remained as an NHS chief executive'. The task was to unify the offices and develop a new strategy for the funds. The pattern of use of the funds was different in each hospital with Guy's tending to favour academic research and St Thomas' giving more focus to service delivery and so it was necessary to create a cohesive strategy and a new merged board of Special Trustees.

A 1998 Briefing Paper set out the new strategic direction as one which needed 'to have clearly stated outcomes on a few major themes/initiatives which can be measured to determine effectiveness and provide value for money'.[44] There was a clear shift to thinking beyond the hospitals to how the funds could help health services across Lambeth and Southwark to be at the cutting edge of clinical medicine and clinical services. Tim and Geoffrey had a much broader and inclusive view of health provision as comprising mental health, community, and primary care alongside hospital services. When support was given for buildings, the bottom line was that the building had to have some sort of charitable significance. With the building of the Evelina, for example, an architectural competition was set up with the Royal Institute of British Architects. The publicity that ensued from the Evelina being shortlisted for the Stirling Architectural Prize in 2006 was hugely beneficial. An arts and heritage policy was established which gave an additional one per cent to support the integration of art within environmental projects as a means of creating a positive impact on patients or staff using the building or services and making them look different to what would have been achieved through NHS funding alone.

Geoffrey and Tim visited endowment charities in New York to see how they got a good outcome from investments. One tangible outcome from the visit was setting up funds to support the development of new ideas. Fundraising was also introduced: 'I think that put quite a bit of grit into the system because if you've got to show people what you're doing externally to get money, it's rather different from having a family attitude to how the endowment fund could be used.' Fundraising for the new Evelina Hospital was the first time that significant fundraising had been undertaken at Guy's and St Thomas'. Another innovation was to use charitable funding to modernise service delivery, and Geoffrey remembers giving sexual health services, stroke services, and kidney disease services £5 million each for transformation projects to modernise services. Kidney disease was 'particularly successful as the clinicians and managers involved in that were broadcasting what they'd done internationally in terms of the transformation and involvement of patients'.

One of Geoffrey's regrets is that a scheme created with the architect, Sir Terry Farrell, to use a vacant patch of land opposite St Thomas' to provide accommodation for health service staff that could be funded by having some private residential accommodation alongside, was refused by Lambeth planning authorities: 'We fell foul of quite a bit of NIMBYism and of parochial things but it would have been one of the most significant things that the Charity could have done if it had come off. The annoying thing about it is that as I cycle past it most days it is a fallow site still. So that was a loss to Guy's and St Thomas'.'

But despite the ambitions of the new strategy, the Trustees remained concerned about Guy's and St Thomas' performance.

> Guy's and St Thomas' should have really been absolutely top. I was never absolutely certain in the 11 years that I was there that we really made the best use of that fund. We tried a number of techniques to try and lever improvements. I often think that we should have been better than we were. Guy's and St Thomas' doesn't always score at the top of all areas of research. In a sense, it should be ticking every single box. It may be now, but I don't think it was ticking every single box in terms of excellence in health service delivery and it should have been with the resource of a charity of that magnitude. Cancer – it really should have been absolutely the top along with many of the best in the world.

One of the factors affecting excellence was attracting top people: 'you do rely on clinicians with foresight to enable it to become great'.[45] When Geoffrey left the Charity in 2009, the magnitude of funds placed it in the top 20 of charities across the UK.

Conclusion

The 1990s had proved to be the most turbulent period in the longer history of the institutions when every aspect of care, research, and teaching was transformed by mergers of one kind or another, driven by external forces. The gains were highly significant and proved vital stepping stones to the further improvement and development of the Guy's and St Thomas' Trust and the merged UMDS and King's in the new millennium. Without these changes it is difficult to imagine that the institutions would have been included in the first cohort of academic health science centres in the 2000s. Nevertheless, it is important not to forget or underplay the many institutional and personal losses through the period, even though with the passage of time the eventual outcomes proved to be highly positive.

CHAPTER SEVEN

Healthcare in the New Millennium, 2000-2010s

Overview

G uy's and St Thomas' Hospitals began the millennium as a combined Trust, continuing to perform a unique role in the make-up of South East London healthcare, as a hospital with national and international reach, whilst effectively serving as a district hospital for Lambeth and Southwark. The senior leadership team was refreshed and worked to address long-established closed and hierarchical cultures to create a more open institution that embraced diversity in every dimension of its work, alongside ensuring financial stability and growth. The decade witnessed significant milestones in the institution's evolvement with Foundation Trust status in 2004, and the establishment of King's Health Partners and an award of an Academic Health Sciences Centre in 2009.

From Trust to Foundation Trust

By 2000 a new senior leadership team was in place. Patricia Moberly was appointed chairman in 1999, with Jonathan Michael joining as chief executive in 2000. Jonathan had trained in medicine at St Thomas' during the 1960s and specialised in nephrology. He had been the first medical director and chief executive of University Hospital Birmingham NHS Trust and in late 2000 was asked to 'put my hat in the ring' to be chief executive of Guy's and St Thomas'. The initial challenges that faced Jonathan were the ongoing post-merger consolidation, and the need for quality improvement across the organisation.

> Guy's and St Thomas' weren't as good as they thought they were so there was an element of complacency. Coming from outside, I had been away from London for 20 years…I couldn't get over how little had changed…they basically needed to up their game which they did…sometimes it takes a new set of eyes to come back and say we can do better.[1]

Patricia too brought a fresh approach compared to previous chairmen. She had lived in the borough of Lambeth since the 1960s and had recently retired from a teaching career. She had a long association with St Thomas' through her public service with Lambeth Council and local health bodies and importantly had experience as a patient. Part of the chairman's job, she said, was appointing excellent chief executives and then looking after them by giving encouragement and support. She took great pleasure in the appointments of Jonathan who served till 2007, and Ron Kerr who became chief executive in 2007, describing them both as 'outstanding' in their roles.[2] One of the early challenges for the new leadership was the progression to an NHS Foundation Trust.

As the Labour Government, elected in 1997, grappled to temper the disruption of Conservative policies with increases in NHS expenditure, conversely the internal market, elements of privatisation and shifts in management culture were cultivated.[3] A ten-year modernisation project – *The NHS Plan* – was published on 1 July 2000, a policy milestone in the development of choice and competition in the NHS.[4] This formalised New Labour's encouragement of the strategic supply of private sector resources whilst committing to continue the tax-based NHS funding system and the free-at-point-of-delivery principle. The subsequent *Delivering the NHS Plan*, published in 2002, set out a new tier of NHS 'Foundation Trust' hospitals. Alan Milburn as Labour's Secretary of State for Health between 1999 and 2003, essentially afforded hospitals Foundation Trust status through new regulatory bodies, rewarding excellent care with further autonomy.[5] The legislation passed by a whisker as there was much criticism of the policy because of fears that Foundation Trusts would create a two-tier system across the NHS and effect privatisation, thereby destabilising the NHS as a whole.

Jonathan had been involved in discussions at the Department of Health building up to the legislation. He was positive about the advantages arising from Foundation Trust status as it increased the 'democratic legitimacy of the organisation' and established accountability to the people it provided services for through the Board of Governors. But Patricia was a passionate advocate for the NHS and had campaigned against the introduction of Trusts in the early 1990s. It was only when Frank Dobson, then Secretary of State for Health, changed the rules around the appointment of non-executive directors by requiring them to live in the area served by the Trust that Patricia had joined Guy's and St Thomas' in 1997. She shared the concerns of many local patient groups and communities about the consequences of change. Jonathan was aware that Patricia was 'politically uncomfortable' with the concept of Foundation Trusts. So in advance of the Board meeting at which, as chief executive, he was going to make a formal recommendation in favour of applying for Foundation Trust status which he knew the Board was very likely to accept, he had to take Patricia on one side to ensure she was fully aware of the repercussions if she voted against the move. For a chairman to vote against a decision that was fully supported by the Board would make the chairman's position untenable. In the event, Patricia supported it and Jonathan reflected that she became 'very effective at running a Foundation Trust with all its democratic opportunities'.[6]

On 1 July 2004 Guy's and St Thomas' became one of the first NHS Foundation Trusts with 800 beds, 9,000 staff, and £600 million income. For some people it provided reassuring evidence that Guy's and St Thomas' had not lost their high standing post-merger.

> Given the then chairman's view about Foundation Trusts and the partly coming out of the NHS and local concern, that in itself was quite a major achievement, and it also said a lot for the governance that the Board and the then Chief Executive had achieved that in a relatively short time.[7]

The creation of Foundation Trusts was seen as a natural evolvement from Trusts, specifically Guy's status as the flagship Trust: 'what started with Guy's has certainly spread out into the start of the Foundation Trust movement. It's interesting it's Foundation Trusts that reintroduced management accounts. Nobody else did, they called it service-line accounting, because they realised, the only way they can create better outcomes and value for patients is by knowing what the outcomes are'.[8] People with longer institutional memories saw the Board of Governors as a welcome return to the pre-1974 period: 'the Foundation Trust is very definitely going back to the governors and much of the autonomy is exactly the same autonomy as the governors had between 1948 and 1974'.[9]

Dawn Hill was the first Black female appointed to the Guy's and St Thomas' Hospital Board, serving as Non-Executive Director from 1999 to 2007 and was a member of the Guy's and St Thomas' Council of Governors from 2009 to 2015. She had been singled out for her expertise in personnel management and nursing experience. When Dawn began her governor role, she felt there were areas of hospital governance that it was difficult to get access to information on such as finances: 'You'd have to dig and ask really, and then they'd say, well you don't need to ask that because the executive directors were dealing with that.' She remembers that Foundation Trust status brought a big shift in governors' responsibilities.

> When it became a Foundation Trust you had to absolutely sit up and pay attention because suddenly it was a different arrangement with the Government, and you really had to know what you were about. You couldn't just swan your way through. As a non-exec now, you really have to know what is going on and be much more alert about what it is that's being done in the hospital. Well, you certainly have to find out a lot more about how the money's being spent and pay more attention to what patients are saying. I think if you're going to be spending the money you really ought to know it's being spent well, and I think that is really important. And as I say, you really have to now know what lies behind decisions, you can't just take recommendations from executive directors and just because it looks good on paper and they give you a right good spin at the Board meeting, that you're going to just accept it; you can't do that.

The role of governors was to represent issues on behalf of patients, staff, and communities, explained Dawn. She described how in her work with the Community Services Committee, she would visit the various community services, and talk to staff to find out what their problems were and whether there were any issues with the services being provided. She would then take that knowledge and understanding back to the Committee so that matters could be addressed.[10]

The successful running of a Foundation Trust in the 2000s depended on the same rigorous business process disciplines that were necessary for running any multi-million-pound organisation. Martin

Shaw, Guy's and St Thomas' Financial Director from 1998 onwards, reflected that the merger had enabled financial efficiencies that allowed development:

> Every five years since, we've built a new building, either on the Guy's site or the St Thomas' site and, you know, that's something that I don't think we could have earned our way into or made sufficient efficiency savings as the two hospitals independently, you wouldn't have been able to generate sufficient funds to do that.[11]

The greater autonomy offered by Foundation Trust status made it a natural choice for Guy's and St Thomas' but they had huge advantage compared to other NHS Foundation Trusts as they continued to benefit from funding from the Guy's and St Thomas' Charity, enabling them to continue to develop sites and services without having to opt in to more risky and costly Private Finance Initiatives (PFI). One of the Conservative policies that the Labour Government strongly advanced was the PFI which was a means of using private capital to fund new hospital building in the NHS. The costs of the design, building, and maintenance would be raised through private consortiums and repaid by hospitals over a long period of years. But private finance cost significantly more than government borrowing, and although arguments were made about the benefits of transferring risk to the private sector, in practice these claims were shown to have been exaggerated.[12] During the 2000s the new Evelina Children's Hospital, as well as other projects including the consolidation of maternity services, were only made possible through Charity support.[13] John Pelly, Chief Operating Officer between 1998 and 2004, commented that, 'one of the things that I think Guy's and St Thomas' has excelled in doing, in fairness, it has some advantages that other institutions don't have and didn't have, is avoid any PFI projects on either side'.[14]

Whilst succeeding at avoiding the pitfalls of PFIs, Guy's and St Thomas' also became effective at growing their commercial arm. Martin Shaw explains how the relationship with the private sector was developed to safeguard their NHS responsibilities.

> We used to take minimal risk but try and generate as much money as we could to help support the provision of more NHS services. We've done a bit in private patients, considering how many consultants we've got, we probably could be doing a lot more, but that's a complex issue in its own right, but we've actually done a deal with the private sector in the building of the Cancer Centre, where somebody else will have space in the building and we'll get the proceeds of that, which will help us make the building of the building viable.[15]

The difficulties of building Thomas Guy House in the 1990s had led to an increased institutional awareness of the challenges of financing, planning, and delivering enormous complex projects. Steve McGuire joined the Trust in 2003 as its first Director of Capital, Estates and Facilities, and played a key role in moving the long history of innovation around estates and income generation forward. The Directorate was set up to improve the physical environment and facilities across the Trust and was renamed Essentia in 2012 at which point it had 1,600 staff and a £150 million annual turnover. The benefits to the Trust from the approach taken by the Directorate is exemplified in the building of the new Cancer Centre which was developed on the basis that the top four floors would be run by a private operator and produce an income stream which enabled the Trust to raise debt finance to build the Centre. It opened in 2016 and hosted the London Bridge Hospital private care patients.[16] As with the Evelina, the Trust held an architectural competition to find the architect for the Cancer Centre and appointed Rogers Stirk and

Harbour alongside developing the innovative funding plan. By 2014, Essentia created a new division – Essentia Trading – which was a wholly-owned subsidiary of the Trust and was intended to take on project management roles for health clients in the UK and overseas. The profits from its consultancy services were to be reinvested into the Trust.

> We learned to design, plan, maintain, and build, so we've got Guy's and St Thomas' into a really good shape. Given we've built up an enormous expertise in-house, we decided to explore the market with other people in the NHS. In terms of external clients, we hope to grow quickly. We can support other NHS clients by offering advice and consultancy, we can advise on construction and health care planning and capital projects. Potentially, we can work with other parts of the NHS and the public sector to help those organisations better understand the estate they've got, to reduce their overheads and to help organisations find solutions.[17]

Opening up the institution

Guy's and St Thomas' continued to serve distinctive communities that had varied profiles in terms of permanence and transience, and health issues. Whilst communities in Southwark and Bermondsey had long roots in the area, Lambeth communities had a high turnover of people moving in and out of the area, and Kennington had a much higher incidence of wealthy households.[18] The hospitals saw a broad range of patients from various demographics from extreme social privilege to appalling social deprivation. Hospital chaplain from 2001, Mia Hilborn reflected that:

> One of the beauties about Guy's and St Thomas' is it's prince and pauper who come in the doors here for medication and

for healthcare issues. You can be from the House of Lords, or you can be a person that's been found around Victoria coach station being sick, you know, drunk, being sick there. You can be…everything comes in, everybody. And I think it was Florence Nightingale who said, it doesn't matter who you are outside, if you're prince or pauper outside, in this hospital you're treated as a prince. And that, I would say, is quite true actually, people are really treated well.[19]

Since the 1990s, as noted in Chapter 5, there was a strong focus in new health policy towards better addressing and meeting patient needs. One example of the ways in which Guy's and St Thomas' responded to the needs of local African communities was in setting up an African Well Women's Clinic in 1997. By the later 1990s, female genital mutilation (FGM) was recognised as an area for urgent improvement in knowledge and communication with the local communities. Comfort Momoh was recruited to begin raising awareness and educate both the community and Guy's and St Thomas' staff. Comfort, from Nigeria, had extensive training, and first heard of the practice during her general nursing training in Lagos. She reflects on the issues surrounding communication and cultural sensitivity:

I came to establish the female genital mutilation clinic – or the African Well Woman's Clinic – before then a multi-agency group was set up, according to what I was told, in 1995–96 because there were a lot of women presenting to the GUM (genitourinary medicine) clinic, the maternity unit, family planning clinic, with FGM related problems; and the doctors, the nurses then didn't know how to approach or how to support women and girls because obviously they looked at it as a cultural issue, traditional issues and they're looking at the sensitivities around that. We don't want to be seen as racist, we don't want to interfere with people's culture and tradition, if you like.

I had to stop and think because the target group, mainly asylum seekers, refugees, and I would say 85 to 90 per cent don't speak a word of English. So, if we're setting up a support service for them here at Guy's and St Thomas' how are they going to be informed, or how are they going to be able to come to the clinic, if we're not having an involvement with the community themselves? So, it was important for me to go out into the community to look for the community. So, I did lots of work, and I know as an African myself that word of mouth is very strong within African communities, so that was the background work we did.[20]

The 2000s marked a period in which Guy's and St Thomas' began to take action to address the discrepancies between the multi-cultural, multi-ethnic boroughs that they served and the lack of diversity in hospital governance. Patricia appointed Dawn Hill, the first Black female, to the Board: 'It seemed to me self-evident that a hospital serving the sort of community we've got, had to have some public diversity on its Board. I remember the last Chief Executive (Jonathan) saying I was becoming a bore about diversity. I said, good, I'll go on boring you until something changes because it's not good enough.'[21] Staff members like Eddyna Danso who had joined St Thomas' in 1989 following her period as a theatre technician at Guy's, had raised questions of representation at Annual General Meetings over many years: 'Why didn't we have a single minority person who's a director? Non-executive, we've now got a few, and when Patricia was here, she started it off... but I think institutional racism is alive and well and going on in the NHS.'[22]

Dawn Hill found the lack of diversity at executive level compared to that at consultant level highly concerning and little changed during her ten-year tenure from 2000 to 2010.

> Amongst the consultant level it's quite different. I mean there's just every kind of ethnicity you can think of. All the best surgeons I can tell you, innovative surgeons are from everywhere else! There's no issue there; all their top people are from just everywhere amongst the medical staff, the paramedical staff, the nursing staff, they've got quite senior people across the board. But there is an issue at the next level about the mix of people, the mix of staff. I don't know how it is now [2014] but when I was there, there was always that issue.

Whilst Dawn and other interviewees cite consultant-level clinicians as a prime example of diversity, the difficulties that clinicians from Black, Asian and other minority ethnic backgrounds encounter in training and career progression has been well documented in the wider history of the NHS and the same patterns are apparent at Guy's and St Thomas'.[23] A consultant who was the first non-white consultant in their department joined the Trust in 2006 and shared their experiences.

> At the interview there was a very senior consultant there, and it was clear that he didn't want me here. It was absolutely clear. He asked very mean questions, and he frowned every time I answered, frowned deliberately to make the rest of the panel notice that he disagreed with my answers. But because I didn't have anything to lose, I was very honest, very straight, very direct, and very relaxed about my answers.

I think it's the fact that I'm a foreigner. It's as simple as that. And in fact, this is not going to be confidential because it's true. When I arrived here, I was the first non-English consultant in this department. It was historically very posh, public-educated English boys and girls. But mostly boys, there was only one girl. So, I think there was a little bit of resistance and there was, there is still, someone in the department who was very unhappy that a non-British consultant was appointed here initially. And they've still been very difficult. I've struggled for eight years with this person. And I know that at the bottom of it is that there's a racism, there's no doubt about that, still.

Well, it's changing rapidly. I mean today [2014] our department is a different story to what it was eight years ago. Fifty per cent of the consultants now in the…department are from different cultural backgrounds. Many of them are born here, but from a foreign background, and they show that they are incredibly qualified. But I think it has also to do with the training. There is still this idea that if you're not trained in the UK, you are not good enough, and I think that's very prevalent still. So, you have to fight harder and show that you are worthy of the place.[24]

Despite decades of experience and excellence in their specialism, this consultant describes feeling 'invisible' during some meetings as colleagues didn't acknowledge their presence. Other interviewees from diverse/non-white backgrounds also recalled discrimination in their recruitment both for training schools and hospital roles. A senior nurse with Jamaican heritage who joined Guy's and St Thomas' in 2011 shared her view that the way to improve the situation was to support people in career development with shadowing and training opportunities to ensure equity. Unconscious bias was identified as one of the strongest influences that needs addressing.

There are lots of things that the organisation is doing to manage that imbalance there currently is around BAME staff not being in senior positions and so I would be speaking out of turn to say that they're not undertaking work, but because of the unconscious bias that exists in our society people tend to choose people who are like themselves; and so if there's a slight difference, regardless of whether it be colour or behaviour or whatever, there's less of an inclination to go towards choosing those individuals. I think the big issue is about people being honest about their unconscious bias.[25]

Studies have also established how staff from Black, Asian, and other minority ethnic backgrounds are often clustered in specialties and/or areas which are unpopular with their white counterparts.[26] Again these patterns held true at Guy's and St Thomas' where most Black nurses worked on the less prestigious elderly care wards and were not represented in senior nursing posts. But whereas the Guy's and St Thomas' workforce was predominantly white, there was a much greater diversity in individuals working in the community.

Within the acute services there is a predominance of Caucasians here; there is a predominance of Black and minority ethnic within our community settings; and I don't know whether that is reflecting about people's greater desire to be in a fast-paced setting where it's – for want of a better word – sexy to be in: as in the acute sector with intensive care, or in A&E, as opposed to being out in the community which is seen as being far more laidback and slow. You're working in patients' homes where it is unpredictable.[27]

Despite Dawn Hill's appointment and the Board's determination to address the lack of diversity in senior appointments, this interviewee found the situation concerning.

As an organisation they are very embracing for differences and for the multi-ethnic workforce that we have; having said that, if you look at our management structure, they are very few, in fact except for our non-executive directors there are no directors within the organisation who are from a Black or minority ethnic background. So that surely must impact on staff in terms of the questioning of the seriousness of Guy's and St Thomas' as an organisation to promote a multi-ethnic workforce, albeit that they are actually doing a lot of work to try and raise the opportunities for all clinicians, all of the workforce, regardless of what their cultural background is.[28]

Though there was little diversity at executive level, the portering department included people from many different ethnic backgrounds. Whilst unemployed in the early 1990s, Bryan Johnson worked as a volunteer at St Thomas' in the portering and transport department. This led to him securing a job and he worked until his retirement in 2011. A Londoner since birth, Bryan had lived north of the river Thames and knew nothing about St Thomas' until he began working there. He spoke of the Trust's zero-tolerance towards racism and the ways in which this became stricter through the 2000s.

I mean, the Trust has always gone out of its way for diversity, and of course, there's zero-tolerance on anyone being racial. There is sometimes, because of the different languages, there can be problems. But we do always have people on site as interpreters, so it's not really much of a problem. No, I think that isn't really a problem. We have zero-tolerance on racism, and I've never really encountered it there at all. There's never been a racial issue there, ever since I've been there. In the portering department, we have, obviously, people of different races, and we get on well together. There's never really been an issue on that, I don't think. Everyone sort of coming from perhaps the south London area, and they all know we're in a sort of diverse area, and certainly, I never had a problem with it myself. We always had people from Africa or the West Indies, and I suppose it's just whoever applies, they pick the best. Obviously, there can be no distinction, so I think it works quite well, that they seem quite hard-working.[29]

Whereas other NHS hospitals had long relied on overseas recruitment to address nursing workforce shortages which had created diversity in staff, the elite status of Guy's and St Thomas' meant they were a highly attractive employer and were in the fortunate position of being able to 'pick and choose' staff. But in the early 2000s, despite the concerted efforts of *Project 2000*, an NHS-wide shortage of nurses existed, which Secretary of State Frank Dobson blamed in part on the emphasis on academic credentials that had put off potential recruits.[30] For the first time Guy's and St Thomas' had to recruit internationally. Patricia Moberly got the Board to agree that they would only recruit from countries where there was a government-to-government agreement such as Spain and the Philippines.

Working abroad to finance their families was common practice amongst nurses from the Philippines where training standards were along American lines – not too far removed from British nursing practice. Christopher Bramaje and Cecilia Saquing had specialised in theatre and recovery work, and described how a group of Guy's and St Thomas' personnel visited their local town to undertake interviews.

It's my first time to be interviewed. And you see professionals, they're well dressed, English people…three people…marking everything that you're saying, so you're like how am I performing? It's so scary for me. But I have to do this. I have to impress them. And then I felt happy that time because they made you feel comfortable during the interview...I think I impressed them because I ended up being hired.

Christopher was reassured to find out that the UK was tolerant towards gay people. He was gay himself and wanted to move to a country 'where I could be free, I could express myself and I'm not going to be afraid'. Many Filipinos went to work in the Middle East but that had a bad reputation for gay people. Christopher and Cecilia took up their posts in 2001 and were the first of around seven cohorts to be recruited from the Philippines for different specialist areas. They remember being well-supported as they settled into their new lives and adapted to language differences and, of course, the British weather. The main difference relating to work was in the everyday use of technology.

> My training was in the countryside, so when I came here, I was happy because we used the machines. Back home we do it manually. Like taking the blood pressure, we had to do it manually, like with stethoscope and things like that. When I came here you just had to connect to the machine, so I was like, oh, it will make my life easier. This is better for me, and you're connected to monitors. We don't have that back home. We don't have all these monitors. So, you will feel the difference, like what does a developed country have with a poor country.

Christopher and Cecilia experienced much less overt racism than earlier generations such as Eddyna had in the 1980s and 1990s, and they found that patients were more concerned about their experience than their ethnicity: 'The moment I say I'm a senior nurse here then they're satisfied' although there have been occasional incidents when patients have joked about being cared for by a group of Filipinos.

When one patient wakes up, he saw all the nurses, Asian-looking nurses, and he told us, am I in Japan, not in England? Because all the nurses looking after me are Asian-looking. And I was like, no, sir, you're actually in the Philippines. He laughed, like, oh, you're joking, I know where I am, I'm in day surgery. I was like, there you go, sir, that's the answer to your question.[31]

Beyond the hospitals, recruitment at the medical schools was widened through the introduction of an access programme that encouraged a wider social range of applicants. The Higher Education Funding Council for England (whose responsibilities have now been split between the Office for Students and UK Research and Innovation[32]) approved an extended medical degree programme. Rick Trainor, Principal of King's College between 2004 and 2014, explained how additional places had been created from c.2002 for students who would not normally qualify on conventional A levels, to give them an extra foundation year and some special tutorial support for the first couple of years of the regular medical course.[33] The annual intake of students on the Extended Medical Degree Programme (EDMP) rose to 50 and drew from low-achieving state schools in inner London. An early study of the programme showed that it was a successful way of widening participation in medicine although it required 'appreciable extra commitment by academic staff'.[34] Cyril Chantler who became Chairman of University College London Partners Academic Health Sciences Centre between 2009 and 2014, views this as a significant legacy of the merger: 'I'm very pleased about the access programme for medical students, so that 50 people from disadvantaged backgrounds are able to enter the medical school each year in King's, who wouldn't have been able to before. That couldn't have been done by King's without the merger, or by Guy's or Thomas' or UMDS.'[35] The access programme anecdotally has also helped with gender balance in recruitment, as Dawn Hill noted: 'I think mostly it's the ethnic minority girls who have taken up a lot of those opportunities. Not so many boys, and Patricia, I think, particularly was behind that initiative, which is very good.'[36]

As discussed in previous chapters, the closed culture of the institutions had long been shored up by old boys' networks with their sports clubs, social dimensions, and hierarchies that shaped everyday practices. Patricia described herself as beginning 'war' on some of these hidden influences that had been at play in the hospitals for centuries including freemasonry.[37] It was well-known that many consultants in London teaching hospitals, including Guy's and St Thomas', were involved with freemasonry and these invisible networks determined appointment decisions and other aspects of hospital life. Mike Messer, who worked as photographer at St Thomas' since the 1970s, remembered that when he was promoted to chief technician, 'I had a couple of funny handshakes from people who came in the department,' and noted that there were photos of the Governor's Hall 'decked out for a masonic meeting with a big, checked carpet down the middle' around 2000.[38] Patricia became aware that freemasonry was influencing consultant appointments.

> When I found out that young doctors were being told quite blatantly that they shouldn't apply here until they were in the Lodge, I'm afraid I took it into my own hands and said the freemasons were not to meet here during working hours. That caused a bit of...they didn't want a female chairman as you can imagine. I asked Jonathan Michael if he was a freemason when he came in 2000 and he said, he wasn't. I explained what was going on and he was very good. Because obviously, as a non-executive chairman, you can growl at people, but you can't actually lay down rules about who hires what rooms and that sort of thing. But he made it very clear it had got to stop, and it did.

As far as I'm concerned, I don't care what they do when they get home, but it wasn't to influence behaviour at work. I'm under no illusions that there probably still is some of it around, but I do think that it's not influencing appointments in the way that it did. I think it stinks actually. Nothing to do with patient care as far as I'm concerned. The main thing was the Lodge meetings were taking place in the hospital, whether during working time or not, I don't know. But they were clearly, if not actually during working time, edging into that. My concern was solely about recruitment and appointments because there's no point in talking about diversity and transparency and all those things if there's a hidden agenda. It's not on. I now ask all Board members if they are freemasons.[39]

Patricia began chairing all consultant appointments herself and the shift led to more women applying and being appointed: 'And of course, women won't put up with that sort of nonsense about trouser legs. Not interested.' In the interests of removing hierarchies in everyday life, she also worked to close the consultants' dining room. It got turned into a senior staff room which Patricia refused to enter because she thought it should be for all staff. However, as new consultants, including more women, joined the staff, and clinical work patterns changed, many brought sandwiches and the old traditions of a formal lunch died.

The natural turnover in staff and new appointments meant that the negative feelings and resistance to change in the immediate post-merger period had generally dissipated. Naveen Cavale, who worked in the Plastics Department sited at St Thomas' from 1997, described how the working environment improved.

There were only five consultants there [in 1997] and there are now 17 and none of them got on at the time. I think

none of them particularly liked working at St Thomas',
they'd all been kind of plonked in as a result of the Guy's
and Tommy's merger or one of them came with the St
John's Dermatology merger or takeover and they were
forced to form a department of Plastic Surgery, they were
forced to work together as an on-call team and share juniors
and so forth, whereas actually they'd been the bosses of
their own little hospitals...I think the atmosphere in the
department has changed hugely for the better because it
was a miserable department to work in at the time and I
almost gave up plastics at the time...they [St Thomas'
consultants] all hated each other, and it was just kind of
Lord of the Flies as far as the juniors were concerned and I
almost gave up at that point. And then actually thankfully
since then I think it has changed hugely for the better and
it's a much nicer department to work in now.[40]

In the late 2000s Patricia sought to draw a line under the merger
fallout and resolve unsurfaced tensions by spearheading an initiative
that became known as 'the truth and reconciliation committee'.
Tina Challacombe who trained at Guy's and became a GP describes
its impact and role in confirming an accurate chronology of events
from every side.

It was a wonderful attempt to get people who were
involved in all those negotiations at the time and right
up to government level, both at Guy's with the Save
Guy's campaign and St Thomas', speaking to all sorts of
commissioners and people in the Department of Health.
It was a challenge to actually clear the air and, in a way,
look at what we've got now, which is actually the strongest
academic and clinical trust in the United Kingdom bar none
and you have to say, would we have got here without that
merger? And the answer is probably, no. So the ultimate

vision that was not shared by everybody has been realised by subsequent very good management in having such a strong Trust and I think the truth and reconciliation was very interesting for all of us to hear the perspective of others, of their recollections of what was going on at the time and confirming things like that I gave to you unaccredited of feeding information to the press, of hearing that confirmed in those sessions was very interesting.[41]

Nevertheless, longstanding parts of hospital life such as the Friends of St Thomas' Hospital and the Friends of Guy's Hospital continued to operate independently and fundraise for the individual hospitals to provide equipment and support the refurbishment of areas. The new strategy of Guy's and St Thomas' Charity stopped the stream of small-scale funding that had supported the hospitals for decades. So although 'huge sums of money were put into a new Cancer Centre which was fantastic, the Charity was no longer willing to provide small donations at the drop of a hat to benefit wards and departments,' reflected Barry Jackson, who became one of the Charity's Special Trustees and has served as President of the Friends of St Thomas'.[42] It was only in 2016 after many years of rejecting the possibility of merging that the Friends joined to become the Friends of Guy's and St Thomas' Hospital, but the time taken to do this meant that it was accomplished without any blood being spilt.

One of Patricia's primary frustrations stemmed from the political context that NHS organisations had to work within.

While I was Chairman I used to talk to junior doctors and say, St Thomas' Hospital has been around for 900 years, and in the 60 years it's been in the NHS, the NHS has already had 35 structural reforms of one sort or another. This cannot be sensible. It's meant you haven't any institutional memory, you haven't had long-term strategic thinking.

In the time that I was Chairman, there were six, or seven Secretaries of State for Health. How could they have had any long-term thinking? They couldn't. They just came and went. [Long-term planning and stability] would have allowed clinical developments to be much quicker and better applied. If I'd known I was going to be here for 20 years with the same Chief Executive, we could have thought about, shall we have a great transplant centre for South London or something like that, that would have taken years to develop. The children's hospital was 15 years in the thinking and planning.[43]

Evelina Children's Hospital

The most notable expansion at Guy's and St Thomas' across the period was the opening of the new Evelina London Children's Hospital on 31 October 2005. The Evelina Hospital for Sick Children was founded in 1869 at Southwark Bridge Road, Southwark. Like Guy's and St Thomas', the hospital was established with an endowment fund; in this case the legacy of Baron Ferdinand de Rothschild whose wife, Evelina, died shortly after the stillbirth of their son. From 1948, Guy's oversaw the Evelina, eventually bringing the children's wards into Guy's Tower in 1973, when the Southwark hospital closed. The wards were named for major benefactors of the original hospital including Rothschild, Arthur Farre and Caleb Diplock.[44] In the context of the Guy's and St Thomas' merger, the Evelina was perceived as a Guy's institution, despite its own distinctive origins. It was located in Guy's iconic tower and included a casualty department and a paediatric ICU. Nevertheless, as the consolidation of services proceeded, the decision was taken to move the Evelina to the St Thomas' site. For stalwart Guy's supporters the changes were regrettable.

They took our children's services, which were also specialist services, and they built a new hospital at St Thomas', the new Evelina Hospital. The Evelina Hospital was ours. It was within the Tower. The one they built was too small. I told them it was too small, and it was too small, and they've had to put more facilities on site for paediatric services. Hopelessly too small. But that all went in the political mix. Great shame. Things can change.[45]

But the paediatricians took the view that, despite their love for Guy's, the most important outcome would be a new children's hospital.

The Evelina became the first purpose-built children's hospital in London for more than 100 years.[46] It took place during New Labour's hospital boom: 26 schemes were built and operational by 2006.[47] But unlike the other hospital projects funded through PFIs, the bulk of the capital for the new Evelina – £50 million – came from the Guy's and St Thomas' Charity with a further £10 million allocated from the NHS. Fundraising was still necessary to complete the transformation of Evelina. Dawn Hill, a non-Executive Director on the Guy's and St Thomas' Board and Governor and Chair of the Evelina Hospital School, explains the crucial role of fundraising in furnishing and equipping the wards: 'The Government had given an amount of money to build the new Evelina, so they had X numbers of money to build it but nothing to actually furnish it and equip it, and that's what the appeal was for, Stanley Fink chaired the fundraising committee and raised all the money, and he's still doing it, raising more money, it's constant for the Evelina and now for the Cancer Centre as well.'[48]

Interviewees involved in the financial administration of Guy's and St Thomas' attributed the successful commissioning and building of the Evelina to their financial autonomy and ability to defy pressure to use PFI. John Pelly, Chief Operating Officer and previously the Finance Director, recalls: 'we were always being encouraged to looked at PFI options and I'm pleased to say that we found a way to resist on every occasion that option, because I'm afraid PFI, in the

NHS, certainly the early wave of PFIs were catastrophically awful'.[49] Martin Shaw, Finance Director at the time, concurred:

> Of the £100 million that we had to do the reconfiguration between Guy's and St Thomas', £50 million of it came from the trustees to build the Evelina Children's Hospital and, in effect, by the time we'd got that planned and we managed to get a signature architect and a construction company together with them taking the risk, but the building cost was £60 million by the time we actually came to build it, but by the time it was built, we controlled the project to time, well, we let the time run over so that the quality and the budget, with fixed price contract, didn't change. So, the availability of trustees' money, good contracting, well thought through transfer of risk to the private sector, on just a construction project, there have been examples of where PFI has worked and, indeed, the University – King's College London – built a building at New Hunt's House on the Guy's site.[50]

The building was designed by Sir Michael Hopkins, who consulted with patients and their families from the outset, devising tools like symbols for each ward to aid wayfinding for the multi-lingual populations of Lambeth, Southwark and beyond. In 2005, the hospital opened with 120 beds and 20 Intensive Therapy Unit beds. Jonathan Michael as Chief Executive of Guy's and St Thomas' NHS Foundation Trust told the *British Medical Journal* that as well as being a 'state of the art hospital', the institution was 'full of imagination, warmth, and fun. It redefines the concept of a children's hospital and will undoubtedly influence the building of new hospitals in Britain and across the world'.[51] The expectation that the Evelina could sway global hospital building trends illustrates the institutional confidence in the wider influence of Guy's and St Thomas', whose reputation as a combined institution was outwardly consolidated in the building of the Evelina.

Kay Lucey had worked as a nursing auxiliary in the specialist milk kitchen in the Evelina since 1991. Her role focussed on providing milk feeds to babies and nutritional support to children, working with dietitians. Kay recalls the importance of their hygiene routines in the milk kitchen, to stave off infection in infants. Taking great pride in her work, Kay helped with the transfer of services to the new site but chose to leave when the Tower wards closed.

> I was involved in the Evelina building – obviously going over and measuring up for everything. It was a wonderful time because everything was new and they were building this marvellous new hospital, the first in 100 years for children and we were involved in it. So, we had to measure up the room and all mod cons and everything. But I still idolised Guy's and I loved it when I went there first, because you were kind of all close together. Because the Tower – we were on the 11th floor, you had the six wards of the Evelina from the top to the bottom and you went around to each one of them. So, you were in very close contact and the difference then when you were going to go to St Thomas's it was going to be a massive, big hospital. Long corridors separated out the staff a lot more, so you didn't have the unit that we were used to working in.

Kay decided that the move to the new hospital was the right point to retire so that 'it was fair for the two girls that I trained up for them to start up new in St Thomas's,' though she continued her Union role as Staff Side Chair for a further year.[52]

Despite all the attention to detail during the planning and design, there were still initial teething problems.

> There was a lot of problems with the building because it's all made of glass. And obviously when the sun come it

didn't open, some of it was opening. Eventually they found
out that they'd put the glass in back to front or something,
but this is years later, after people sizzling inside there. But
they're still very warm in that building.[53]

The overall design was driven by a desire to create the best possible
environment for child patients yet staff found many aspects added
difficulties to their work. The curved corridors were intended to
allay fears of children yet from a porter's perspective, these made it
trickier to manoeuvre beds through the space.[54] Not being able to see
beyond the curves led nurses to feel under pressure to be in two places
at once.[55] Staff focus groups also revealed that the design created a
sense of 'over-familiarity' in the hospital which led to parents tending
to 'over-rely' on staff to look after their children whilst waiting for
treatment. They feared that if there was an accident, the parents
would hold staff responsible.[56] Reflecting on the different 'feel' of
the old and the new Evelina, Kay described feeling an intimacy and
connectivity within the old Evelina, even though it was situated in
the tallest hospital tower in Europe, compared to the new hospital
which was 'massive' with very long corridors. Yet despite the scale
of the new Evelina, by the early 2010s there was a sense that the
building was 'too small'.[57]

The Evelina Hospital was a significant moment in the wider history
of Guy's and St Thomas' but it also exemplified the deep changes
surrounding the care of children that had taken place through the
lifetime of the NHS. Whereas in the 1950s children were not given
access to their parents whilst in hospital, by the 2000s it was a matter
of course that parents were a vital part of their child's care. Daily
routines included children being dressed in the day and having
schooling. Cyril Chantler reflected on the changes.

> Children are not little adults, they have their own emotional,
> physiological needs, they suffer from different diseases,

they have to be managed in a different way, you can't look after adults as though they're children, but you can't look after children as though they're adults. At it's very simplest, if a child is sick, they need their mother or father or both alongside them. The paediatrics that I grew up with, the parents weren't allowed in the hospital except during visiting hours and the trauma these children suffered, is a matter of record, which went on to the rest of their lives, so it was really important for us, that the experience that these children and their families were going to have was the sort of experience they get in a good children's hospital like Great Ormond Street, not that you would get in the children's ward of an adult hospital run essentially for adults. Most hospitals in the country now provide children's services for children, not for little adults, they have children's casualty departments, I mean, it's improved immeasurably.

What do children need when they go into hospital, if they're in for any length of time? They need to continue to be educated, so you need a children's school and children to get dressed every morning, because life has to go on as before, I can never understand why the first thing you do when you're sick, as an adult, is they take your clothes away from you, well, why do they do that? I mean, often put you in gowns which are indecent, why do that? Children in hospital have their clothes, they get dressed and they spend their day like that and in the evening, they have a bath and go to bed and have a story and go to sleep, a bit like home.

In a health system where most patients are elderly with chronic disease, there is still a danger that children can be marginalised. 'I think the current generation of paediatricians are just as alert as I used to be, but things are much better than they were,' reflected Cyril.[58]

Ensuring children had continuing access to education was a further facet to care at the Evelina. Soon after the hospital was established in the 1940s, a school was set up to educate patients. The school is currently classed as a Department for Education hospital community special school and is funded by the London Borough of Southwark for 68 planned places, with children numbering up to 80 per week. The pupils are either inpatients at the Evelina, siblings of inpatients or occasionally regular outpatients. Dawn Hill, Governor and Chair of the Evelina Hospital School, recalls how bewildered parents were when schooling was offered: 'they look as if you've gone completely mad'.

> So, you have to really explain to them what the school does and how it works. The staff are really very well trained in how to approach teaching in a hospital school; it's not the same as the school down the road, it really isn't...Like with everybody, you don't spend a long time in hospital. But there are children who have heart and neurosurgical complaints and spend a long time in hospital and attending the school. Those unable to leave their beds are taught at their bedside. The renal children are attached to their machines three times a week; the school is their main school. They are at a main school, but they spend less of their time there and more time in our school.[59]

The school environment is created for patients through integrating the education into hospital care; whilst most children are taught in classrooms in the atrium of the school, those unable to leave their wards receive bedside support.

Mergers and identities

The merger of UMDS with King's brought immediate benefits as recounted in Chapter 6. But meshing institutional identities to create

Guy's, King's and St Thomas' proved to be a longer and trickier process. The 1990s had brought the merger of the United Medical and Dental Schools with King's College London, creating three new schools: the Guy's, King's, and St Thomas' School of Medicine, of Dentistry and of Biomedical Sciences with formal completion in 1998. As Guy's and St Thomas' consolidated the merger of services across its two sites, academic teaching was also reorganised, with Guy's becoming the primary campus. Whereas the UMDS merger involved only medical and dental students, the UMDS and King's merger included students from all the schools spread across medicine, dentistry, and biomedical sciences as one faculty within a multi-faculty institution and the high student numbers made it difficult to establish a collegiate atmosphere.[60] Incoming students were no longer applying to distinctive institutions, yet on arrival they needed to distinguish themselves from other university students. The name of Guy's, King's and St Thomas' was rapidly reduced to GKT and the GKT name became welded to student identity. Robert Lechler, who became Dean of the merged school in 2004, explained:

> Students…consciously apply to King's College when they're choosing their medical school; they don't apply to GKT. However, once they are here, I mean very soon after they are here, they develop this very strong allegiance to the hospitals and their traditions, and the student community is very wedded to this GKT title – Guy's, King's, St Thomas'.[61]

One of the initial GKT cohort, Jawahar, recollects the transitional period:

> I think they were in the process of re-branding everything to King's College London, but still, half the stuff still said Guy's and St Thomas' Hospital Medical School, or words to that effect. So…and because I played a lot of hockey, it was drummed into me that I went to GKT, I didn't go to

King's College London. And that's still how I feel. If people ask me where I trained, I tend to say GKT, then I wait to see if they actually know what that is, if not, I have to say King's College London. But no, I think there still definitely is a rivalry between the...basically, the London Bridge Campus, which is GKT, and the other two, Waterloo and the Strand, there still is a rivalry.[62]

Likewise, Lewis Moore applied to read medicine at King's without any understanding of the hospitals and their history, and 'how they have this sort of separate history to the university'. He was introduced to the GKT traditions through recruitment to the sports teams.

The first time I heard the term GKT, was when I was approached by rugby players in the bar, who wanted to recruit me to their team, and I said, what's GKT? And they sort of looked aghast and explained to me how different we are from those at the Strand, and those pursuing pure scientific or academic careers. And obviously my involvement in the GKT, because that now is very much aimed at the membership of the health schools, rather than King's College, as a whole.

Lewis also acknowledges the role of place in his sense of GKT based at Guy's.

We all have our lectures here at Guy's in the Greenwood Lecture Theatre...certainly all the sports teams and all the medics tend to drink in Guy's Bar, here at Guy's, and the rest of the King's College London students tend to congregate over on the Strand, and there's a bar over there. I feel like it probably contributes quite a lot, particularly when the buildings themselves are so historic, you get a real sense of identity from the Keats statue, as I mentioned, Thomas Guy himself at the front…yes, the air of history of the place is quite enticing, quite romantic.[63]

But GKT proved problematic at institutional level as it detracted from the King's broader brand and in 2005 the name was changed to King's College School of Medicine, sometimes followed by Guy's, King's College, and St Thomas' Hospitals.

> The renaming caused concern amongst students and graduates, as issues of the *GKT Gazette* record. Controversially, the 'ban on GKT' extended to sports teams, who were renamed as King's College London Medical School (KCLMS) sides – even though around half of their players were from outside of the medical school. In 2013, the former GKT clubs became known as KCL (Medics), but later that year a motion was passed in the Student Council to change the official title of the sports teams back to GKT.[64]

In 2014 King's College London decided to rebrand itself as King's London and released a statement saying that the Medical School would be known as the GKT School of Medicine at King's London. The intention was to communicate the institution's autonomy along similar lines as its rival, University College London, which by then was using UCL. Students objected vociferously to what some of them saw as the 'pretentious' rebrand of King's and pushed King's management for a further statement about the name of the Medical School. On 7 January 2015 Robert Lechler released a statement saying, 'We have agreed to embrace GKT in the name of the School of Medical Education. The full name will be King's College London GKT School of Medical Education and will come into effect immediately.' The plans for the King's rebrand were dropped.[65]

Simon Cleary joined King's College as a student in 2010, studying on a joint honours course in physiology and pharmacology. He had been attracted by the 'friendly' feel of Guy's campus. When interviewed in 2014, he was studying for a PhD in pharmaceutical sciences.

> I think that a lot of people are conscious of the history, and there are good reasons for people to accept that the hospital campuses are now part of a bigger institution, and it makes things more efficient and, sort of, amps up our global standing. But it's difficult to do that without, sort of, losing a friendly collegiate environment and respecting the history of the institutions that became one with King's College London. But I don't think a particularly bad job's been done of that. I think the GKT thing is quite nice, in that it includes or has come to include a lot of people – medics, dentists, nurses, biomedical scientists, and perhaps physios, and dieticians and midwives, though I've not seen that many of them; which I think is part of why people have campaigned recently to change the official names of the hospital sports teams back from KCL medical school to GKT, because it more accurately reflects what the teams are. At the same time, I think that GKT was another kind of cumbersome acronym that replaced UMDS. And although it's quite a good description, it's difficult from a sort of branding perspective, now that GKT isn't really a thing anymore, because it isn't the GKT School of Medicine or Biomedical Sciences. I think a lot of newer people who are coming in see GKT as a bit old fashioned and weird. And you can hear it in people's attitudes from Imperial and UCL who are…well, maybe Imperial, who think that it's a bit old fashioned that the medical students still refer to themselves as something that hasn't been around for a good decade or so.[66]

The bedding down of students within GKT was relatively unproblematic compared to the process of relationship building between the Trust and the College.

The Trust and the College

Great care and attention had been taken during the UMDS and King's merger, to ensure clarity and fairness, particularly with regard to the ownership of properties and the 'intricate division of labour' in research, teaching, and clinical care whereby many employees of the Schools were honorary consultants in the hospitals, and many consultants held honorary positions in the Schools.[67] A body known as the Continuing Trustees of UMDS had been set up with the intention that this would safeguard the risk of UMDS properties acquired by King's being sold off for purposes other than education and research. Despite these efforts, in 2002, a proposal by King's College Council to sell off Block 9 caused a public outcry. The Block 9 section of St Thomas' included the premises of the old St Thomas' Hospital medical school and adjacent buildings and was transferred to King's College as part of the merger with UMDS. Over time it became little used as the Medical School transferred many of its operations to the Guy's campus. In 2002 King's College Council received a bid from the Aga Khan, world spiritual leader for Ismaili Muslims, to set up a museum for Islamic art and culture. The proposal caused a public outcry and a Save Block 9 campaign began which obtained over 10,000 signatures for its petition and staged a protest across Westminster Bridge. Kevin Burnand, Professor of Vascular Surgery at St Thomas's, said, 'it would be a disaster for us and the NHS if this land was lost. I and many of my colleagues would chain ourselves to the railings in protest'.[68] The Council argued that they had a responsibility to make best use of resources and the Aga Khan's bid was for between £20 million and £24 million whereas that from Guy's and St Thomas' Charity on behalf of the Trust was much lower at £10.5 million.[69] Patricia Moberly recollected vividly the day that the Chairman of King's College London Council visited her to tell her of the intention to sell the site: 'it was only by causing acute embarrassment to the University that it wasn't sold'.[70] The episode left a blight on the relationship between the Trust and the College, but it also acted as a catalyst for collaboration on a new scale.

Rick Trainor took up his post as Principal of King's College and Professor of Social History in 2004 after serving as Vice Chancellor at the University of Greenwich. On arrival he experienced the negative effects of the 'residual tension' from the land sale debacle but also recognised 'unrealised potential' in the collaboration between the College and Guy's and St Thomas'.[71] Shortly after Rick was appointed, he was joined by Robert Lechler who became Dean of the Medical School. A specialist in transplant medicine with research interests in transplantation immunology, Robert had spent most of his postgraduate career at Imperial. Like Rick, he had been attracted to King's because he saw it as 'something of a sleeping giant'. In other words, it was 'underperforming' compared to its potential and he saw an opportunity to build and shape something significant. The underperformance was attributed to a mixture of factors including a lack of ambition, not enough distinguished academics, a lack of coherent leadership, and an 'under-developed relationship' between the University and the hospitals: 'so they were courteous to each other but did not seem to recognise the symbiotic relationship that a university and its hospital partner need to have if they are going to achieve the impact that they can'.[72] Rick and Robert worked in different capacities to rebuild the relationship.

> A big effort was made by [Robert Lechler] and other colleagues in the Health Schools working closely with Jonathan Michael, who was then the Chief Executive of Guy's and St Thomas', to achieve a more positive set of results around the relationship between the College and the Trust. There may already have been a bilateral sort of

liaison committee, but it was certainly beefed up and made more regular. Robert became the Deputy Chair, not just a member, but Deputy Chair of the Board of Guy's and St Thomas' and I started up a series of one-on-one meetings both with the then Chairman of Guy's and St Thomas', Patricia Moberly, and with Jonathan Michael. That carried on subsequently with their successors, Sir Hugh Taylor, and Sir Ron Kerr.[73]

Through these endeavours which included agreeing that there needed to be a shared decision around the future of the Block 9 site, came a growing recognition that the effective combining of research, teaching, and clinical care resources across the College and the Trust would produce new opportunities. Thus the strengthening of the bilateral relationship was the process that laid the groundwork for serious discussions about the development of an academic health sciences centre.[74] In 2006 Robert was appointed Vice Principal in charge of the five Health Schools within King's – medicine, dentistry, nursing, psychiatry and biomedical science – and two years later he was appointed to lead King's Health Partners in the creation of the new academic health science centre. Proof of the strength of the collaboration and the creation of a shared vision came with the award for a biomedical research centre from the National Institute of Health Research around 2006. King's were on the verge of declaring themselves an academic health sciences centre when the Department of Health intervened with a competitive accreditation process. The development of academic health sciences centres was one of the recommendations in Professor Sir Ara Darzi's review of London health services in 2007.[75] King's Health Partners was formally accredited as one of the UK's first Academic Health Sciences Centres (AHSCs) in March 2009.

Robert reflected on how King's Health Partners met the criteria for AHSCs:

I would say that in order to be an internationally competitive AHSC you need three basic criteria to be fulfilled: you need quality and excellence in all three domains of the tripartite mission, so that's the clinical services who deliver the research that you prosecute and the education that you deliver, and I think we can safely say that we have all three. Secondly you need breadth, and we provide almost a comprehensive range of clinical services, bearing in mind the inclusion of the South London and Maudsley. We have a very broad research portfolio in biomedical research, and we have probably the broadest education portfolio of any UK centre because we train doctors, dentists, psychiatrists, physiotherapists, dietitians, pharmacists, so there are very few health professionals we don't train. So those are the basics but the thing that excites me is then the range across which innovation can be developed, and so if you think of it as a spectrum we go all the way from whizz-bang, gizmo-orientated research where we're developing novel diagnostics and therapeutics, built on basic science, engaging in first in human studies in patients and so on, all the way through to novel models, and novel modes of delivering healthcare and evaluating those latter innovations.

Robert drew on an example of a care pathway for homeless patients to exemplify the direct benefits to care arising from AHSC networks.

It turns out that St Thomas' A&E department has the highest incidence of homeless attendees of any A&E department in the UK. These patients cost eight times as much as a non-homeless patient because of all the social complications around their complicated lives and they tend to have drug/alcohol abuse problems and mental health issues, and so we've brought this multi-professional team together to address, to sort of zone in on these patients when they come into hospital and deal with all the aspects of the issues that these patients, and it's absolutely fantastic, and I am immensely proud – even though I've had nothing directly to do with it – that we're doing that. That is absolutely appropriate activity for an AHSC, particularly because it's going to be coupled with evaluation, so you evaluate any innovation in order to learn from it and then if it turns out to be a valuable innovation then of course, it's our responsibility to disseminate that information. And there again we have another opportunity created by the birth of the AHSC – the network – because our AHSC covers the whole of South London, and that is a vehicle to adopt and disseminate innovations as we generate evidence that they are valuable.[76]

Notably, the award of the AHSC preceded a final decision about the future of Block 9 as it was not until 2012 that agreement was reached to refurbish and redevelop Block 9 and the Prideaux Building for a mix of medical education and office use.[77]

The AHSC was viewed as an extraordinary achievement that had not been anticipated a decade earlier and was only made possible through the UMDS and King's College merger.

The final outcome…which I think [former Dean] Ian Cameron and I would have thought was probably not possible, which was that ten years later, King's would be an academic health sciences centre, I mean, after all, there are only five in the country…Manchester, Cambridge, King's, UCL and Imperial, and after all the medical schools in England, those five were deemed to have a level of science at a capacity and achievement to justify being an academic health science centre and that King's should be one of them is amazing. When you think where we were in 1998 when the merger came together, much of that is due to what my successors and Ian's successors have done, but it wouldn't have happened if we hadn't gone down that route.[78]

Conclusion

By the end of the 2000s the turbulence, unhappiness and disarray caused by the mergers of the Guy's and St Thomas' Trusts and UMDS with King's College had largely settled. 2010 marked the centenary year of Florence Nightingale which was celebrated across the Guy's and St Thomas' community. In October 2010, the Evelina Children's Hospital marked its 5th birthday with a fancy-dress party for children and the launch of a new fundraising initiative called 'Superkids' by Guy's and St Thomas' Charity. Over its first five years, pioneering work at the Evelina included widening a valve in a child's heart by an MRI scan rather than X-ray, and a kidney transplant involving the removal of hostile antibodies from the child's blood before the transplant had continued. The Evelina also continued to care for thousands of local children and offered continuity of care from child to adult services. The successful establishment of King's Health Partners, externally validated by the award of an Academic Health Sciences Centre in 2009, also gave evidence of Guy's and St Thomas' ability to thrive as a merged institution. Patricia Moberly's reign came to an end when Sir Hugh Taylor took up his appointment as Chairman on 1 February 2011. Sir Hugh had a very different background with a civil service career and senior roles in the Department of Health. The institution he took over was visibly different to the one Patricia joined in 1999 with the new Evelina and the King's Health Partners giving the institution an external watermark of excellence. Speaking at the Annual General Meeting of Friends of St Thomas' Hospital in May 2011, Sir Hugh said:

When paperwork and bureaucracy get to me, I go for a consolation walk around the hospital and see so many examples of human kindness as well as medical advances which even ten years ago would be regarded as miracles. What gives this hospital its edge is that not only does it employ many gifted people but has the wonderful support of the Friends and Volunteers for which we are most grateful.[79]

CHAPTER EIGHT

Communities of Care: Changes and continuities since c.1970

Overview

T he final chapter concludes by discussing the changes and continuities in the everyday work and experiences of students, patients, and staff since the 1970s. It reviews how Guy's and St Thomas' has maintained strong connections with the past despite the profound transformations across many aspects of institutional life and healthcare, and thus counters traditional narratives of radical linear change across the NHS. Guy's and St Thomas' heritage is shown to be a vibrant and embedded influence across Guy's and St Thomas' which has the capacity to promote resilience and constancy to core values in the face of external flux and change.

Working environments

Across the period, the everyday and often invisible work around patient care and service delivery continued, but one of the most notable differences from earlier times which affected all aspects of working life and institutional processes and systems was the integration of technology and digital communication systems. The so-called 'Millennium Bug' in 1999 at the turn of the year 2000 which threatened to cause computer errors because of having to reformat calendar data was alarming. Kay Lucey, nursing auxiliary at the Evelina, in her role as a union representative, reflects:

Basically, every computer had to be checked. You had the cardiac machines; you had a mass of things. It was a massive thing had to be done. Thank God nothing happened...I mean that was brilliant because nothing went down, but I mean it was a fear. Because if you were going in for an operation, you'd think, my God, I hope they're not doing it in 1999, wait until the Millennium Bug is over. But no, but everything went fine. But the preparation for that was massive, a lot of staff had to look into all the different things.[1]

Porter Bryan Johnson's work was improved by the introduction of new electrical beds that were 'much bigger' than the smaller, manual beds, and only required the press of a button to raise and lower them. But he noted how moving these larger beds through corridors and spaces that were not designed for beds of this size led to 'a few problems, especially getting into certain lifts. Literally some of the new beds won't go into certain lifts'.[2] And as noted in Chapter 7, Filipino nurses Christopher and Cecilia were struck by the way in which technologies were integrated into every aspect of patient care when they arrived at Guy's and St Thomas' in the early 2000s.[3]

Mike Messer's work as a chief photographic technician also changed dramatically with the introduction of Microsoft PowerPoint software that enabled academics to produce their own teaching and presentation slides. Mike had worked at St Thomas' from 1970 and his role varied from photographing the student experience, sports events and so on, to post-mortem photography for lecture slides, images to be published by academics, and production of teaching slides. He had already resisted the closure of his dark room for developing film on the basis that camera film produced greater precision in images. The darkrooms at Guy's and King's had been closed in the 1990s. Around 2000 Mike found that his slide production services were no longer required and the usual autumn rush to produce teaching materials in advance of the new term abated. When the Photography Department was disbanded in 2007, Mike performed a central role in creating an historical record of St Thomas', providing negatives that were matched with medical school records by Rosieanne Pinnie. These were archived at the Gordon Museum. For almost 40 years, Mike had witnessed change across the various facets of hospital work and whilst in post he held the institutional visual memory.

One of the key changes in working practices was the introduction of much greater sensitivity and regulation around the handling and photographing of human remains.

> That changed drastically, there were no rules when we started so some would come into the department with a bucket almost steaming away with a placenta in it which had just gone out from a birth and you'd put a bit of paper down and you'd slap it on and take a photo, bits of leg, bits of anything used to come in. But then rules started to be introduced that you had to have a separate room, with a separate basin and taps and that, well, that really killed it. So what you had to do was go to the post mortem room or go to the laboratory where they were doing the research and photograph it there.[4]

Foundation Trust governance structures brought new opportunities for staff and patient engagement and in 2006, Bryan joined the Trust's Members' Council as a staff member.

> Other people suggested that I could try for it, they seemed to think I'd be good at it, and I quite enjoyed it. We had various meetings and it's quite interesting to hear what was going to happen. You just felt more a part of the hospital. We even had to vote on the new chief executive which I thought was a bit of a privilege.

Bryan's expertise in portering enabled him to contribute that perspective to site developments. For example, when Gassiot House was refurbished in 2008 to include a new outpatients' department, the expectation was that patients would arrive at ground floor level by walking over Westminster Bridge as there was no vehicle access to this level. Bryan, however, was aware that many patients would arrive either by car, or transport at the lower ground level and would then need portering. His concern was that there was no effective shelter on the ground floor and patients would need to be taken in wheelchairs across a main car park: 'I've done it, but it can be a bit of a worry.'[5]

In staff groups apart from consultants, staff turnover had risen since earlier decades partly due to the changing nature of work where individuals would encounter new opportunities, noted Kay Lucey. For many years, staff had been rewarded with a silver medal for 15 years' service and a gold medal for 25 years' service that was presented at a special event, hosted by the Chairman. By the 2000s, Kay reflected that as it was now unlikely that people would remain at the same place for 25 years, the Staff Side were looking at other items for rewarding service such as certificates or sets of glasses that were not too expensive.[6]

Cultures of care

Alongside these visible markers of change, other shifts were more subtle but equally significant including the moulding of behaviours and attitudes to better reflect the emergence of a more egalitarian society. Hierarchical working cultures, driven by the professional norms of medicine and nursing had long shaped staff-staff interactions. When Kay Lucey joined Guy's in 1991 as a nursing auxiliary, she found that the senior nurses 'looked down' on the more junior nurses. Because she loved Guy's she decided that she would work to change the culture and became involved with the

Union, becoming Staff Side Chair by the time of the merger. This work resulted in the establishment of a new relationship between the Union and the Trust, with the Trust accepting that the Union's motives were driven by the aim of establishing equality for all its members: 'by the time we finished we had a partnership agreement which is a big thing for unions and a Trust to have'. One of the things Kay is most proud of in her long career was: 'getting the low paid trained up, acknowledged, getting them changed from the opinions the way people thought of them, that was one of my best jobs. Because I thought nowadays, everyone talks to each other and acknowledges that we're all human beings, not that she's down there'.[7]

From 2005 with the appointment of Eileen Sills as Chief Nurse there was a concerted effort to 'close the gap between "the board and the ward" and increase the senior nursing clinical visibility' so as to improve patient experience and quality of care. Fridays were designated as days when senior nurses would return to work in clinical departments: 'You have to go and see what it's really like if you are going to effectively lead and be a voice for your staff and your patients.' This initiative extended into weekly meetings to discuss quality of care issues which became known as a 'safe in our hands' briefing. It also developed benchmarking practice by identifying examples of excellent or poor practice on wards and using those as a means of learning. In 2012, the film 'Barbara's Story' was released which followed the patient journey of an older person with dementia and by 2017, 10,000 out of 12,500 staff had watched the film and engaged in discussion.[8]

The culture of nursing had lost many of its hierarchical aspects since the 1970s and Georgina Day, who joined the Florence Nightingale School of Nursing and Midwifery, King's College in 2010 to train in nursing, described a much more informal and friendly working relationship with teaching staff: 'We still have a lot of respect for them, because they are incredible people, but you see them a lot more than I suppose you might have and they are around, which is good.'[9] *Project 2000* as recounted in earlier chapters established an academic base for nurse training which created a very different experience for student nurses compared to earlier generations who had trained in the Guy's and St Thomas' Nursing Schools. Yet the initial shock of acclimatising to work on the wards remained. After an introductory period of classroom teaching from September, Georgina went on the wards in early November and found it a daunting experience.

> You'd have cases that would be very harrowing, and I think with every nursing student, I know there was a lot of tears and School were really supportive with that. They were really good to encourage us to accept that those were feelings we would feel. There's a lot of death going on out there, there's a lot of people in really bad situations and really struggling and I think that's very hard to deal with, especially I suppose when you're a bit sheltered and you haven't seen people really struggling with life and then you come up here, up to London, and you see that not everyone has it good and that some people's worlds are just falling apart. It's very, you know, it's very hard to take as an 18-year-old that you can't do everything for these people, I think that's one of the things I struggled with most, I think.[10]

Betsy Morley who had trained at Guy's during the 1950s reflected that academic ability was not always a portent of an excellent nurse who could truly care for patients. During interviews with nursing applicants, she describes herself being at odds with the nursing tutor who focused on A' Levels, whereas her concern was that potential trainees should fully understand the realities of unsociable hours and strict uniforms that they might not think particularly suited their appearance. She remembers how important support from other student nurses was during training. Living in the nurses' home meant that once nurses went off duty at night, they would meet up for cocoa or a drink.

> If one of us had had something that really affected us, whether it was that we'd really had a problem with the sister in the sense that she'd really wiped the floor with us and we'd found it very upsetting, or that there'd been an untimely death on the ward we were working on, you could talk it over, and that was a saving grace in so many instances I think at that time. I'm not sure what they do now. I mean if you are a single parent and you've got two little kids, you can't go home and start telling them what's happened. So, I'm not quite sure how much they have to bottle that up.[11]

The introduction of day surgery and the huge reduction in length of patient stay produced a much higher turnover of patients, and this reduced the time that nurses had to build relationships. As ward sister, working up till the late 1990s, Betsy Morley began each day by going round the ward to say 'good morning'. That enabled her to identify any issues that needed addressing so that the patient could be put at ease and would recover more quickly. Georgina reflected on the importance of establishing relationships with individual patients and gaining their trust as this had a direct effect on how they responded to being asked intrusive things, and they became 'a lot more compliant with the things that you need to achieve with their care'. At the outset, she treated patients formally, calling people 'sir' but rapidly realised that patients wanted a different kind of relationship that enabled them to feel comfortable with a nurse: 'They always want to know a bit about you, because you take every aspect of their life, and you analyse it. They often ask, Nurse, what about you? Where are you from? Do you have siblings? That's a perfect example of them wanting a bit back from you so it's a mutual thing.'[12]

The establishment of an academic base for nurse training increased tensions around its status as a vocation and/or a profession.[13] 'I don't think you can be taught to care,' noted Georgina. She had met people who had always wanted to nurse, whereas she had discovered through her training that caring was an intrinsic part of who she was. Florence Nightingale's heritage at Guy's and St Thomas' was both a positive and a negative factor. Students continued to reference 'Florence' in their everyday exchanges and jokes and 'idolise' her to some degree, but the historical stereotype of nurses as a 'handmaid' to doctors was not helpful when nurses wanted to be recognised as 'a modern, dynamic, enthusiastic workforce'.[14] Yet the core values of nursing appear as strong as ever in Georgina's perspective.

> Nursing is an incredible career, it makes you happy, it makes other people happy, you get to do so much for other people that can go some way to improve their experience and I think that's very important to me. I'm not going to make them well, I'm not going to cure them of everything that's going wrong in their lives, but if I can…for that temporary time that they're with us, if I can make something a bit better, that's great. Like, today I found a lady a pillow and that sounds so stupid, but that was important to her, because she was uncomfortable and it was distressing her, it was worrying her that she'd had a really rubbish night, but by finding her a pillow and a vase for her flowers, I think she saw that people cared and people were there for her as she started her time in hospital, so that was, I think, yeah, you can help people.[15]

In 2014, Georgina who was then in her third year of training, won an Outstanding Contribution to Practice Placement Award at the Student Nursing Times awards.[16]

In medicine, stereotypes of the consultant as 'God' coloured the treatment of patients in the earlier periods and several senior clinicians reflected that from the perspective of the 2010s, the historical treatment of patients was problematic.

> Looking back, I think the patients weren't treated in the way we like to treat them now. For instance, the consultants would come and use their surname: how are you today, Thompson? They were all lined up in the ward with the sheets all carefully aligned, and sometimes they would have a blackboard in the middle of the ward, the Nightingale ward, where it'd be completely quiet. No one was allowed to talk or anything. Everything's prepared for the great man to come round with his students. And we thought it was fantastic. But basically, they were treated as objects. I'm not saying everyone wasn't trying very hard. The nurses looked after them extremely well. They did everything that they could. But in terms of the quality of care that I think the consultants offered, I think it was below what you might have hoped in retrospect.

One of the dangers produced by the glorified status of consultants was that when they 'undoubtedly made errors and there was no one to criticise them or to talk about it they didn't necessarily advance'. Richard Thompson describes as a junior doctor having to create a separate prescription chart so that a patient could be given a low salt diet and keeping it hidden from the consultant because he did not believe in the therapy.[17]

As a paediatrician, Cyril Chantler was prompted to think much more carefully about communicating with patients and the need to address the imbalance in power. He recounted a conversation with

Ian McColl, Professor of Surgery at Guy's until 1998, who served as Parliamentary Private Secretary to John Major between 1994 and 1997 and then became Shadow Minister for Health between 1997 and 2000.

> Ian McColl said to me, you know, I've learnt a lot from being involved with the children in Guy's. I said, good. He said, for example, I've learned that it's really important that when you're talking to a patient you should sit down so you're the same height as them and not just stand above them. So now, every time I go around my ward, the adult ward, I always make sure there's a stool I can pull out and sit down on it so I can talk to the patient. I said, very good, Ian. I'm pleased you do that. The other thing you should do is take your trousers off. He said, what? I said, well, if you really want to have a proper conversation with somebody so that you can actually deal with them in a way which they'll feel comfortable and there isn't a power relationship between the two of you, then you'd better get undressed, because they're undressed and how do you think they feel lying like that semi-naked and you're in your suit and your white coat? I said, the other thing you could do is allow them to get dressed. He said, why don't we do that? I said, I've no idea, I'll ask Matron. She said, we'd lose the clothes! I said, Oh for goodness sake, we don't lose them on the children's ward, why would you lose them on the adult ward?[18]

Humorous though this anecdote is, it demonstrates how a much greater clinical awareness of the nuances of patient interactions has developed over time. Cyril explained how the complexities of modern medical treatments create a context in which there are multiple risks and benefits to interventions that require deep consideration by the individual patient and their families.

I mean, things have moved on, that was a long time ago, but it gets more and more important, because nowadays people have to make choices. I mean, modern medicine can be very difficult, can be very dangerous and it could extend your life at a hell of a cost, so the people who have to make the decisions are the patients and their relatives, so the doctor is there as a supporter and adviser who is like the navigator. The pilot is the patient, so you've got to find ways of making sure that they are really well informed and can make decisions which they're not pressurised in any way into making, for whatever reason. So, some of this stuff may sound a bit silly, but it actually is very important.[19]

Reconfiguration of medical training systems has also supported a more open culture that includes patients. One of the mechanisms which reinforced consultant status was the 'firm' system of medical training whereby medical care was led by consultants, supported by trainees of varying seniority and long hours were spent in the hospital. Helen Lawrence joined St Thomas' in the 1980s as executive assistant to Stephen Jenkins, then District General Manager. Her parents ran a pub in Waterloo through the 1950s and she remembers it being known in St Thomas' as 'Ward 13': 'I'm going to Ward 13, said staff, and then if the person they wanted was out at Ward 13 they'd ring the pub and ask them to return.'[20] From the trainees' perspective, when the firm system worked well it provided excellent professional and emotional support and enabled clear lines of responsibility for patient care. From the 1980s, multidisciplinary team approaches were introduced as part of a broader push to address the increasing complexity of medical treatments which involved a broad range of health professionals in discussions about patient care.[21] In 1993, the General Medical Council published *Tomorrow's Doctors* which set out a new framework for medical education with broadened curricula and a range of assessment-types.[22] Through the 2000s the firm system began to fade with the introduction of *Modernising Medical*

Careers, a new programme for postgraduate medical training and full compliance with the European Working Time Directive in 2009 which limited excessive hours of work.[23] Many of the retired senior consultants interviewed for the project expressed concerns that these new ways of working have diminished the support systems that were a vital part of their own training experience.

Patient experiences

A greater awareness of the patient perspective across Guy's and St Thomas' and the need for patients and families to be fully involved in discussions around care is one of the key shifts from the 1970s to the 2000s. Medical care of patients broadly raised few issues. The basis of complaints revolved around patient-staff relations, particularly attitudes to care and poor communications and often highlighted wider issues across the NHS.

After retiring from nursing, Betsy Morley took on managing complaints from 1998 to 2009 and noted how the number of complaints rose over the period with a designated department established to manage the complaints process. She attributes the rise in complaints to the way in which society as a whole has developed a blame culture: 'everybody complains about everything. It seems to have got out of control'. She took what she described as a 'nursing approach' to handling them.

> Say out of 20 complaints, perhaps three of them made my hair stand on end because I realised something awful had gone wrong with the care, the rest of them were just complaints that they didn't like the food and so on. When I was a ward sister, all we ever got were lovely thank you letters. If I got a complaint that rang completely true of somebody who was totally distressed, I'd immediately pick up the phone and ring this person and say, my name's

Betsy Morley. I'm a complaints officer. I've just read your complaint and I am so sorry. And the response, nine times out of ten was fantastic. Thank you so much for ringing.[24]

But some patients had poor experiences and found the bureaucracy involved in making a formal complaint was too much. In 2002 Cathy Ashley went for a routine mammogram and was called back for a biopsy which diagnosed cancer. She was treated with a lumpectomy and lymph node clearance and stayed on Hedley Atkin ward. The breakfast room floor was not vacuumed and, in the washrooms, she saw blood on the wall: 'there seemed to be never anybody in there to clean it off'. She found her treatment to be so traumatic as to cause flashbacks and the hospital arranged for her to get psychotherapy and aromatherapy from the Richard Dimbleby Cancer Support Unit. She refused radiotherapy treatment as her research had shown it was more likely to cause heart trouble and when a further lump appeared in 2005, she tried homeopathy before agreeing to take Letrozole, an aromatase inhibitor. This shrank the tumour which was removed surgically and after remaining on Letrozole for a further five years she was clear of cancer and only required monitoring through regular mammograms.

Several months after Cathy had undergone her second lumpectomy in 2006, her husband, Ray, developed leukaemia. He was offered a blood stem cell transplant which had a 50:50 chance of success. One of his siblings turned out to be a perfect match so the transplant was done but Ray took a long time to recover. In 2010 he developed graft-versus-host (GVH) disease which happens when particular types of white blood cells in the donated cells attack the body's cells because they see them as foreign. Because it was in his gut, one of the side-effects of GVH was incontinence, but it was only when Ray developed diabetes and needed insulin injections that Cathy was able to get the district nurse to visit. When she asked the nurse about how to manage the incontinence she was told, 'Oh, that's not a priority.

We only deal with priority things and incontinence isn't a priority.' Ray's condition sadly deteriorated and his last stay on the Samaritan ward was not smooth. After losing his mobile phone a few months previously whilst in hospital, he lost his iPod and was no longer able to listen to the jazz music he loved. The Ward Manager was sympathetic, but the iPod was never found. When Cathy visited in the afternoons, she found that Ray was covered in food after feeding himself lunch because his condition made his hands shake. His bed was in an isolation room and faced a blank wall so he asked for the bed to be turned around so that he could look out of the window. But this meant that he was under the air conditioning and as the staff could not control the system, he became very cold because he insisted he wanted to look out of the window. Ray asked to be transferred to Lewisham Hospital so that it would be easier for Cathy to visit, and he eventually died there.

When asked in her interview what the hospital could have done to have improved things, Cathy mentioned individual members of staff who had been wonderful but most of the issues resulted from poor communication and little effort to support patients and carers in the gruelling business of treatment. Talking to other patients and carers in the waiting room, Cathy found that her experiences were common.

> We were all struggling with what we were having to cope with. And I think a bit more about the problems of graft-versus-host disease should've been made available to us earlier, so that we could understand what we could have to face ... the side effects of the drugs were so horrendous, they were changing Ray's personality some of the time.

This reflects Cyril Chantler's earlier observation that the benefits of new treatments are not without high cost. It was also a period of building works on Guy's Tower where the day unit was situated.

Cathy and Ray arrived one day to find the entrance had been moved because the front of the hospital was being renovated. The usual car park was not available, and Cathy had to drop Ray off and get a porter with a chair to transfer Ray to the day unit or the clinic, then move the car to the NCP car park and return to find Ray. She had been given no information about alternative places to park, or how to reclaim the costs.

> It turned out that the hospital had a fund to apply to for that and nobody told us. So, we weren't being given information that we ought to have been given information about, and I don't know who should've been responsible. But I do think those sorts of things could've been done much, much better.

She also had to make sure she brought all the tablets and incontinence pads Ray would require if he was told he had to stay in because otherwise it would be impossible to get the required medicines from the pharmacy in time. Lewisham proved to be a more supportive environment.

> If as a carer you said something, somebody would try to get something done, whether it was one of the doctors or one of the nurses. And I mean sometimes I thought the nurses were run ragged, but they would somehow point me in the right direction. The PALS (Patient Advice and Liaison Service) people were visible. They had someone on a desk as you walked into the hospital. The PALS people at Guy's were in an office that you couldn't get into.[25]

Cathy and Ray's experiences illustrates how in the 2000s, despite the extraordinary advances in treatments it seemed much more challenging for staff to pay attention to the details that made such a difference to patient and carer experience than it had been in earlier decades. Formal structures were in place such as the PALS and there were patient/carer support groups, but these were not easy to access, and Cathy was so busy with trying to look after Ray on a daily basis that she did not have time to engage with these. Staff pride in the cleanliness of wards also seems to have diminished, in part because of the change in nursing structures and cleaning rotas being more fragmented. In Lewisham Hospital Cathy spotted blood on the side of Ray's bedside cabinet and when she asked the cleaner who was mopping the floor, the response was, 'I don't do blood, that's the nurse's responsibility'.

Outsourcing had been introduced into the NHS from the 1980s but Patricia Moberly reflected that when she took up her role in 1999, catering and cleaning had been brought back into the hospital as there was 'now a very strong feeling that these are better done by staff'. Staff in these roles were generally low paid but were motivated to work in the hospital by public sector values and their sense of community. As staff members they developed a much stronger sense of allegiance to the institution.

> I expect people when they're walking down the corridor and they see some poor old lady who doesn't know the way, to stop and help her and if necessary, take her there. You may well say these are soft values, not hard values, and efficiency and the bottom line are more important. But soft values are much harder to develop and much easier to lose. It's very important hospitals have that quality of staff involvement.[26]

Francis Tibbles had a long association with Guy's and St Thomas' as he had kidney dialysis in the 1960s and then had a successful kidney transplant as covered in Chapter 3. More recently his parents have been cared for in hospital. Speaking in 2012, he reflected on the differences in care over time.

When I've been on wards when my father and mother have been in hospital it seems to be so much more of a rush. The other thing, I definitely noticed when my mother was ill in St Thomas' – admittedly she had dementia by then – I have to say I was disappointed by her care. I know it's difficult with a patient with dementia, and they've got lots of things on, but I would often come into the ward and find her completely uncovered. Her food was just sitting there. While I know they're busy, I didn't expect that from St Thomas' nurses. I didn't think that was the care that she deserved ... when I looked at the nurses, they seemed to be from a totally different culture than they were then. It's nothing to do with ethnicity or race or anything like that. It's more to do with the fact that it seemed to be, I don't know, sloppy. When you were on those wards in St Thomas' [in the 1960s and 1970s] everything seemed to be cleaner, smarter, and not untidy. At some point it seems to me that some of the standards have slipped, and I can't put my finger on why that is. Whether that's coming from management at the top in the nursing structure. Whether that's coming from consultants having less say of what's happening on those wards or not bothering so much about that side of things.[27]

Yet Francis' experience as a renal patient is excellent: 'I've only got to go up to Guy's, ask to see a consultant and they'll deal with it.' A commitment to making patient experience of the highest quality in every aspect of Guy's and St Thomas' work shines through many of the interviews despite the difficulties in achieving this consistently. Ron Kerr became Chief Executive of the Trust in 2007 and stressed the importance of framing patients as consumers to the present day.

If I'm honest there are different ways in which you need to get involved with different patients, and some people are expert patients. Often patients with long term conditions are as expert as the clinicians who are treating them and know exactly what they need and are really clear about that. Other patients are less so. Although many people don't like the notion of patients as consumers because they think it sort of demeans the business that we're in and what healthcare's all about. I actually accept and support that point of view. But whatever language you use the concept of being a consumer in terms of being the person who is clearly always right in the sense that what they're comfortable with is what we should be comfortable with, and that they've got a right to know about what's going on and be involved in what's going on, that concept is only going to grow and we've just got to get used to it and make sure that Guy's and St Thomas' are at the forefront of that sort of movement going forward.[28]

Notably many staff express greater confidence in the care offered by Guy's and St Thomas' than in other hospitals.[29] For example, chaplain Mia Hilborn describes the case of a colleague, whose mother received a late diagnosis and poor cancer care elsewhere. When transferred to Guy's and St Thomas', the patient was given palliative care that extended her life by one year.

She had the best care that anybody could ever hope for. And that was the reason why her daughter brought her to Guy's, to the cancer wards at Guy's because she knew she'd been mucked about by particular problems in a different hospital. They took it to a full complaints process. But she wanted the best care she could get for her mother, and that's why she brought her here. And you'll find a lot of staff do that, they bring their loved ones here when things haven't gone so well.[30]

Part of staff confidence comes from the notion that the high academic status of the institution produces higher clinical standards. One interviewee had trained dentistry in the 1960s and later specialised in prosthetics at Guy's Dental School before going to work in Hong Kong. On his return to the UK, he had a bad hip and visited a consultant at Ipswich Hospital. He asked which prosthesis was used and when told it was the stainless steel and polyurethane one, he said he wanted the titanium one 'because what you call orthopaedic bone cement is actually very similar to the polymethylmethacrylate that we make denture bases out of and what do you do if the patient is allergic to it?'. The consultant had not heard of anyone being allergic to it and told him that as his hip was not 'too bad', to come back when it got worse. After realising that it was possible for him to ask for a referral elsewhere and after doing some research, the interviewee asked to be referred to David Nunn at Guy's and St Thomas'. Based on the same X-ray David said, 'oh, that's quite bad, we'd better get you in reasonably soon if we can'. The operation went smoothly and there have been no problems since. David Nunn became ubiquitous in 2011 for shouting at the then Prime Minister David Cameron and Deputy Prime Minister Nick Clegg during a visit to the orthopaedic ward when he believed they had not followed the guidelines on infection control. The interviewee sent David Nunn a letter saying, 'what a pity that didn't happen when I was there because there'd have been two of us shouting at him'. Comparing his experience with those of elderly relatives receiving treatment at other NHS hospitals, he believes everybody was more caring at Guy's: 'Guy's has this specialist breed at its core which encourages people to take responsibility and to do things properly for the sake of the institution.'[31]

The quality of consultant appointments lay at the core of Guy's and St Thomas' capacity to continue to develop as an excellent institution. Patricia Moberly reflected that the most exciting aspect of her role was the appointment of excellent clinicians with the capacity to further develop innovation and quality in services.

> The strength of the big teaching hospitals is they are rooted in very poor and deprived communities where people have access to a very good health service, and they're very proud of it. And on top of that, you've got this very specialised stream of work and the two need to be hand in hand, in my opinion. If you have a big patient population, there's lots of interesting diseases that very clever doctors will want to look after, but then they will also develop things that are so unusual that people come from all over the world to benefit from them. And that is a very important balance. I remember sitting here one week, appointing somebody who was an expert in a new technique for removing stones from your salivary gland. And I think there were only two or three people in the whole of Europe who do this, and people were coming to Guy's from all over Europe to have this done. Very proud of them, very impressed. Would you want to spend your whole life thinking about salivary glands? No, but thank goodness somebody does. Next week, I'm, sitting here. What am I interviewing for? Somebody who is an expert in the tear duct. I was absolutely astonished at the skill that person had. He probably knew more about tear ducts than anybody else in the country. Really, you learn something every day. These people are absolutely amazing. And if you're attracting that quality of clinical care and research, then these places will maintain that reputation, but you've got to be thoughtful enough and adventurous enough, and supportive enough, for them to want to come and do that work here, otherwise they'll go and do it somewhere else.[32]

Death and faith

Amidst all the changes, death remained as much part of hospital life as it had always been. Bryan Johnson described how carefully the porters managed the moving of a body after death.

> That's always been a job of two porters, it's a rather delicate matter when we take the removal casket or box onto the ward. We have to draw all the curtains so none of the patients can see us. The body's already wrapped, of course, but we have to transfer that onto the special trolley, and convey it to the mortuary, and put it in the fridge. As well, out of hours, when the mortuary staff aren't there, the relatives sometimes come along to view their relatives. And what that's involved is removing the body, the patient, to a special viewing chapel, which is very nice, and putting it on a special trolley and just uncovering the face and covering the rest, because it's in a shroud, with a special quilt or blanket. But the worse is when you've got children, of course. Not a very pleasant thing to talk about, but obviously, it's got to be done.[33]

Christian faith practices had been embedded in the institution since the earliest times with morning and evening prayers on the wards supported by regular Chapel services. Whereas these daily rituals stopped through the 1980s and early 1990s suggesting a diminishing in the place of faith in hospital life, from the late 1990s onwards the merged chaplaincy 'burgeoned' as it rose to the challenge of offering support to patients and families across faiths and denominations. Chaplain Michael Cooley reflected on the closeness of hospitals to life: 'birth and death and coping with illness' and because 'religion is how we handle, cope with, live our lives, the two are bound very close together'. He described Guy's and St Thomas' as a community with 'an openness to religious faith whatever form or structure that takes'.[34] The chaplaincy expanded significantly during the 2000s to support Guy's and St Thomas' increasingly diverse patient and staff communities. Dundas Moore, a retired GP who volunteered as a chaplain at the Trust, reflected on the breadth and depth of services available to patients and their families.

> We have every denomination and every faith that you can think of. We have the Muslim chaplain, we have the Hindu chaplain, we have the Jewish chaplain, we have all the denominations of the Church of England chaplains, we have the Methodist. You name it, we have it. In general, it works out that you're responsible for a ward and you visit those people who ask for a visit. The reception you have from the nurses is very good, and especially at the weekends. I've done it for 13 years now and I really cannot recall a hostile reception from a staff member. And they'd be perfectly entitled to say, look, we're busy, we can't be, you know, bothered with this sort of thing. So, there's a nice, mutual respect between staff and the chaplaincy. Mia Hilborn [head of chaplaincy] is very strict on making sure we do all our mandatory trainings. We have a study day, if not two study days a month; we have marvellous retreats. We've been to Caldy Island in Wales, to Rome, to Assisi, we went to Avila in Spain, all sorts of wonderful things. It's a very unique set-up here and we have a terrific respect for each other. And if the nurse says a Muslim patient would like to see somebody, you go and see them and then you say, I'll get your priest to come and see you.[35]

Dundas remembered a young Japanese woman who suffered from heart disease collapsing. She was Buddhist and within an hour the chaplaincy team was able to find an appropriate chaplain to give support before she died: 'this is the sort of facility we offer 365 days a year, the team are on call for the whole of that time. And that sort of example just illustrates how unique and amazing it is'.[36]

The interweaving of faith with hospital routines is exemplified by the multi-faith prayer room that gives the Muslim community of staff and patients space for daily prayers. Omar Mahroo joined Guy's and St Thomas' as ophthalmic clinical lecturer in 2011 and testifies to the strong connection between work and faith: 'We're here to worship God and worship isn't just about direct prayer or ritual practices but also caring for the sick, as with other religions, and trying our best to alleviate suffering. My faith gives me a spiritual meaning to my work so I directly feel it influences me.' Taking five minutes out to pray gives time for reflection: 'often I come out with a fresh thinking about a particularly complicated diagnosis'.[37]

Not only were local communities diverse in and of themselves, but Guy's and St Thomas' continued to have a stream of Muslim patients coming from countries in the Middle East including the United Arab Emirates, Qatar, Saudi Arabia and elsewhere. The chaplain often became an intermediary who could explain the Islamic stance on various topics. For example, in the case of a Muslim patient whose condition was worsening, and the medical team suggested withdrawal of treatment.

> The reason the family were not happy with this was that their understanding was this was something that was wrong from an Islamic point of view. I was called upon and after understanding from both sides we came to a conclusion Islamically it is allowed because there's more harm being done than good by letting the treatment carry on. After this consultation the family were more at ease in terms of making that decision. As a chaplain we never ever try to overwhelm a family or a patient to take decisions but

would always give the choice and let them make the final decision or you know just make it easy for them to make that decision.[38]

By the end of the 2000s faith seemed as fully embedded in hospital life as it had been in earlier centuries and the chaplaincy was responsive to keep expanding to meet the needs of new communities, for example, Black communities with Pentecostal faith. Chaplains described being involved in multidisciplinary team meetings, bringing Guy's and St Thomas' values of care into sermons and providing teaching on Islamic medical ethics for the medical curriculum. Alongside the creation of multi-faith spaces and the celebration of festivals like Eid and Diwali these initiatives have served to make faith a visible and integrated part of daily life.

Kinship bonds

John Bibbings worked at St Thomas' from the 1970s, first as Group and then District Catering Manager. He reflected on the deep bonds between staff and institutions.

> Each person that's either worked in Guy's or St Thomas's has left a little bit of themselves in that hospital and to join them together is a very challenging thing to do. I joined St Thomas's family, part of me is still here, I don't think if you've worked here for any length of time you ever lose the association with St Thomas's and it's a lovely place to have worked. It was a nice family and each family looked after its own and it's a shame now that that's going to change but it will take a generation and a half at least to bring together.[39]

It is notable as mentioned earlier, how the sense that Guy's and St Thomas' operate like a family cannot be understood solely as a nostalgic reflection of retired staff as it is manifested by the new generations.

> I think I'd see Guy's and St Thomas' as one organisation. My office is here at St Thomas', and we still have some part of women's services at Guy's, the colposcopy and all that. I just see both as a big family, if you like, rather than separating them. Maybe at the beginning it's like, oh, Guy's, St Thomas', but now you get used to it, especially with the shuttle bus running regularly you can hop in, hop out, and go to Guy's, come to St Thomas'; to me it's like a big family.[40]

> I feel like it's family now because we've been here for a while. I've bonded, so most of them I consider them very close to me. So, the relationship is better for me. It's like a family actually.[41]

> It's like we are a close-knit family here. We've also been here for a long, long time, so I don't find any difficulty dealing with our colleagues. Managers, they come and go.[42]

The intensely strong bonds created between place, people, and cultures are as evident in those who spent their whole careers at Guy's and St Thomas', as those who worked there for a matter of a few years. Continuing involvement post-retirement with the institutions is facilitated by alumni organisations including the Friends of Guy's and St Thomas', and the Veterans' Association. Wendy Mathews trained in physiotherapy at St Thomas' in the 1950s and went on to work in the Physiotherapy Department on research led by John Mathews, Wendy's husband, who was consultant in rheumatology. After retirement, Wendy researched the history of the naming of the wards across Guy's, St Thomas' and the Evelina Hospital since their origins, publishing *My Ward* in 2009.[43] The book speaks to the deep associations with particular wards held by patients receiving care, and staff working in those places and the ways in which wards are microcosms of the identity of the hospitals at institutional level which act to bind patients and staff to particular places and cultures.

Helen Lawrence who had worked at St Thomas' since the 1980s, left in 2001 but returned to run the Veterans' Association which had begun in the early 1950s and was a social network for people who had left St Thomas'. It was open to anyone who had worked there for ten or more years and was informal without status or titles, just first names and surnames. Once a year a lunch was held, preceded by a service in the Chapel. But despite the rules that no one could reserve seats for the lunch, 'they will break legs to get into the dining room first to be able to sit with their group. It's that family feeling again. They want to be back with the people that they worked with, shared life with'.[44] One interviewee remarked how the experience of working with colleagues at St Thomas' in the 1960s was so formative that it had created an unbreakable bond that had remained strong and vibrant, despite the fact that the group never again worked in the same organisation.[45] Eddyna Danso joined Guy's in the 1970s and despite difficult experiences of discrimination and her ongoing concerns about racism in the NHS, she has forged deep connections that she wants to maintain beyond retirement, even to the point of wishing to have her memorial service in Guy's Chapel. One of Eddyna's motivations for contributing her experiences to the project was to speak for colleagues she had worked with for decades but had sadly passed away. She spoke warmly of a deep relationship with a member of the catering department who had brought food up to theatre who had died unexpectedly around 2010. Her passing was marked by a memorial service in Guy's Chapel which was well attended by all who knew her. This event caused Eddyna to reflect on the fact that after retirement she would like to continue her relationship with Guy's and St Thomas' through Union work and alumni networks.

I just feel connected to that place. I can remember coming for my interview, meeting great people and them being really supportive, and just treating me like I was a human being, not like I belonged to any categories. The people I have worked with, it's what's kept me going. The staff nurses when I was on permanent nights. The sisters, who I know are not with us anymore. But they supported me, and I couldn't have done it without. When, you know, you are a single parent, you are rushing to get children to school, rushing to do a job. I'm sure I wasn't always 100 per cent, but you felt that there were people who were supporting you, watching your back for you...When I go, I would like my memorial service to be at the Chapel.[46]

Past, present and future

So, what does this history suggest for the future of the Guy's and St Thomas' Foundation Trust? The social value of historical institutions such as Guy's and St Thomas' is significant. They hold a pivotal place within local communities and the nexus of healthcare. At their best, they are a positive force for social cohesion. For patients, staff, and publics, these communities are deeply connected by their collective commitment to care. Throughout the period, care has been the constancy: patients have fallen ill and needed admission, babies continued to be born, and death was a regular event within hospital walls, though rarely taken for granted. As many of the voices in this book remind us, the care of the sick and vulnerable have remained at the heart of Guy's and St Thomas' however much patient needs may at times have been muffled by the outlying turmoil and turbulence of wider political and social reforms. This collectivist way of working together for a clear purpose has been severely challenged and weakened on occasion, particularly by the upheavals of mergers and wider changes across healthcare. Yet the metaphor of 'family' holds fast to the present.

Generations of staff and patients from the 1940s to the present describe their experiences of working, training, and/or being cared for at Guy's and St Thomas' as being part of a family. The concept of what 'family' has meant at different times has been redefined and renegotiated to reflect wider changes in society and culture, in a similar way to which social understandings of 'family' have shifted from a close, tight unit to a wider, blended configuration.[47] The persistence of 'family' as a metaphor for these experiences suggests that despite the many alterations in the processes of delivering care and the changing notions of what 'good' care looks like at different moments in time, the shared experience of providing care has inspired a purpose that has united past and present generations, binding them together irrevocably. This purpose has been the positive force enabling staff to overcome old institutional rivalries and external challenges to be broadly subsumed through the emergence of new, blended cultures of healthcare. At national level, NHS policy pays little attention to the social value of historical institutions like Guy's and St Thomas' or notions of public interest and service, even though Guy's and St Thomas' close political connections frequently place them at the vanguard of policy development. Yet it is these social values that have underpinned the resilience of Guy's and St Thomas' communities in surviving and thriving during the decades of change since they became part of the NHS in 1948.

Change over the period has been complex, ongoing, and unpredictable. Like other NHS organisations, Guy's and St Thomas' have had to weather a barrage of externally imposed political change, although they have at times been protected from the storm to varying degrees by recourse to endowment funds and political influence. One of those times was the initial period in the NHS between 1948 and the 1974 Reorganisation. This brought no great change to Guy's and St Thomas' – direct reporting lines to the Ministry of Health coupled with their political connections and financial capacity enabled the institutions to maintain their autonomy in vision and purpose.

The shift to embracing responsibility for the health needs of local communities during the 1960s, for example, was as much self-driven as a response to external influences. The period between 1974 and becoming Trusts was the most fraught and volatile in terms of constantly moving goal posts and financial stringencies. The 1974 Reorganisation of the NHS meant losing Boards of Governors and new local reporting lines, both of which made the institutions vulnerable to the wider pressures and changes across the NHS, especially around the funding cuts driven by the wider retrenchment of welfare state provision after the global oil crisis of 1973. There is no doubting the shock of having to work within externally imposed frameworks and the appointment of commissioners to take over the AHA at the end of the 1970s exemplifies this perfectly. From this point onwards, Guy's and St Thomas' became more proactive about anticipating and negotiating with change. For example, action was taken to embark on a merger between Guy's and St Thomas' medical and dental schools to create UMDS in 1983 rather than wait for the imposition of a merger with an institution that might be more problematic. The slow and considered implementation of the merger allowed people to adapt to the idea of change in an organic fashion. Yet there was no way of avoiding or pre-empting the consequences of the reconfiguration of London health services in the 1990s through the Tomlinson review. The Government's introduction of Trust status in advance of the reconfiguration intensified these difficulties – both Guy's and St Thomas' had had to undergo a challenging period in advance of applying for Trust status to convince staff that this was the right decision and there was no indication at that point that such major change was on the horizon.

The enforced merger of the Guy's and St Thomas' Trusts in 1993 created unprecedented disruption to institutional identities and the redevelopment of services across two large sites. The emotional toll on staff was enormous. Many were not able to tolerate the changes and left. Those who remained had to work through a very difficult period and it took well over a decade for the Trusts to settle into new patterns of services and site configurations to be completed. The merger of the Trusts and the way in which the process caused them to compete for primacy was the lowest point in their centuries-long history that was deeply destabilising. The knowledge that further mergers of medical and dental schools were likely to be imposed led to Guy's and St Thomas' initiating the merger between UMDS and King's College. Despite the lengthy, complex, and painful processes of merging training schools and becoming part of a multi-faculty institution, this merger is still regarded as a much more positive event because it was initiated by the institutions themselves.

The political context of the NHS has been one of the biggest challenges for the institutions over this period. The present system means that governments operate as short, politically determined time blocks during which successive Secretaries of State for Health seek to make their mark. This environment is not conducive to the strategic and long-term planning that is required to establish high quality health services that meet the needs of patients and embed innovation. It has been an ongoing source of frustration for both clinicians and managers who know that much more value and progress could be realised beyond the confines of the political pull and push which constrains longer term thinking and planning.

National policies have though been just one strand in this history. Other strands include the enormous change in medical knowledge and technologies that have revolutionised the treatment of previously fatal conditions like cancer but also stretched institutional resources to the limit. Nor are new treatments without risk, and this has created new dilemmas for patients needing to choose between various options for treatment plans. Demographic change with ebbs and flows in populations, alongside a growth in ethnically diverse communities have required services and approaches to flex; Guy's and St Thomas' have responded to new patient needs such as establishing services for FMS and developing a multi-faith chaplaincy. The workforce has also become more ethnically diverse but, as has been the case across the NHS, racism and discrimination have been a core part of the experiences of ethnically diverse staff. Guy's and St Thomas' have made sustained efforts to address these difficult issues and things have improved markedly across the period, but it has still been a struggle to establish diversity at the most senior levels of leadership in management and nursing. The appointment of Avey Bhatia as Chief Nurse in 2020 was notable as one of the first NHS appointments of a chief nurse of Asian heritage.[48]

Since the 1980s, the marketisation of the NHS has been driven by the political need to contain costs and this has propelled the past decades of neoliberal reforms. One of the central dissensions in current debates on the future of the NHS is its status as a public sector institution which operates as a quasi-market. Yet this polarisation of public and private ignores the longer history of institutions that pre-date the NHS and the ways in which this longer history has shaped their periods as NHS organisations. Guy's and St Thomas' have been defined by their former histories as voluntary hospitals and have continued to enjoy generous endowment funds that have provided development opportunities on all fronts, from research to buildings, from patient care to staff support. Throughout the period, charity and independent fundraising has continued and there are enormous numbers of volunteers who contribute to hospital life on a daily basis. Caring for the sick and the vulnerable has not precluded Guy's and St Thomas' from being early adopters of business techniques, building shopping malls, and funding the building of new treatment centres through selling space to private enterprises. Their history as independent voluntary hospitals meant that they did not baulk from engaging with modern business and management approaches to better develop and improve services and infrastructure. The history of Guy's and St Thomas' is the sum of their individual and merged histories which are defined by much longer traditions and influences than the 75 plus years they have spent as NHS institutions.

Guy's and St Thomas' rich, long, and now blended history has emerged as a powerful source of resilience and comfort during times of externally imposed challenges. History has proved a valuable resource for creating positive narratives to make sense of change and provide reassurance during turbulent times. On joining the NHS in 1948, Guy's and St Thomas' individual histories supported their strong, positive self-identities as players on a global scale with significant international standing. The narrative around the UMDS merger portrayed the process as a return to the eighteenth-century origins of Guy's and St Thomas' as the United Hospitals of the Borough. Exchange schemes and research collaborations widened institutional perspectives and during the financial stringencies of the 1980s, Guy's clinicians turned to their US counterparts at Johns Hopkins for inspiration. Wyndham Lloyd-Davies contextualised the 1990s' pressures on clinical budgets in the history of St Thomas' since the fourteenth century.[49] Though at times such positive self-belief may have led to complacency and an over-exaggerated sense of achievement, it also provided the wherewithal to survive difficult periods. Guy's and St Thomas' resilience to change and challenge is exemplified in the emergence of the positive and dominant narrative which establishes the successive mergers as stepping stones to the establishment of Guy's and St Thomas' NHS Foundation Trust as a leading provider of healthcare, education, and research, with the connections to the Academic Health Sciences Centre used as a hallmark of quality.

Across Guy's and St Thomas' sites, current staff and patients encounter past generations and institutional history made visible through statues, plaques, portraits, and most prominently through the Florence Nightingale Museum. Physical spaces, objects, rituals and social networks bind the past to the present, creating a vibrant sense of the longer history of Guy's and St Thomas'.[50] The knowledge and understanding of where the institutions have come from and what has been achieved to date, permeates the everyday work of caring for the sick, training health professionals, and delivering health improvements through producing new medical and scientific knowledge to underpin interventions. It gives current generations the resilience to withstand new changes and challenges, and, in this way, the history of Guy's and St Thomas' retains its vital influence on both its present and its future.

Endnotes

Chapter 1

1. Guy's and St Thomas' NHS Foundation Trust. (n.d.). *Mary Seacole statue unveiled.* [online] Available at: https://www.guysandstthomas.nhs.uk/news/mary-seacole-statue-unveiled [Accessed 18 Aug. 2023].
2. Guy's and St Thomas' NHS Foundation Trust. (n.d.). *Five south east London NHS trusts join forces to tackle long COVID.* [online] Available at: https://www.guysandstthomas.nhs.uk/news/five-south-east-london-nhs-trusts-join-forces-tackle-long-covid [Accessed 22 Sept. 2023].
3. Guy's and St Thomas' NHS Foundation Trust. (n.d.). *Guy's Tower regains title as world's tallest hospital building.* [online] Available at: https://www.guysandstthomas.nhs.uk/news/guys-tower-regains-title-worlds-tallest-hospital-building [Accessed 18 Aug. 2023].
4. Day and Klein's study of the evolution of the Department of Health identifies a shift in career patterns amongst civil servants in the Department by the late 1980s with a growing number 'seeking experience in the NHS.' P. Day and R. Klein (1997) *Steering but not rowing? The transformation of the Department of Health: a case study*, Bristol: Policy Press, p.32. See also S.L. Greer and H. Jarman (2007) *The Department of Health and the Civil Service: From Whitehall to Department of Delivery to Where?* London: Nuffield Trust.
5. S. Snow (ed.) (2011) *The recent history of Guy's and St Thomas', 1970s to 2000s: Witness Seminar held at Guy's and St Thomas' NHS Foundation Trust on 16 June 2011*, University of Manchester: Centre for the History of Science, Technology and Medicine.
6. A. Portelli (2018) 'Living Voices: The Oral History Interview as Dialogue and Experience', *The Oral History Review*, 45(2), pp.239–248.

7 A. Thomson (1999) 'Anzac Memories: Putting popular memory theory into practice in Australia', in A. Green and K. Troup (eds) (1999) *The houses of history: a critical reader in twentieth-century history and theory*. Manchester: Manchester University Press, pp.240-1. See also G. Currie and A. D. Brown (2003) 'A narratological approach to understanding processes of organising in a UK hospital', *Human Relations* 56(5) pp.563-86; Y. Gabriel (2000) *Storytelling in Organisations: Facts, Fictions and Fantasies*, Oxford: Oxford University Press; D. Ritchie (2014) 'Top down/bottom up: using oral history to re-examine government institutions', *Oral History*, Spring 2014, pp.47-58.

8 W. G. Ouchi (1980) 'Markets, Bureaucracies, and Clans', *Administrative Science Quarterly* vol 25 pp.129–41; H. Reeves (2018) 'An Exploration of the "Railway Family: 1900–1948', unpublished Ph.D. thesis, Keele University.

9 (1973) *Accounting for Health: a report of a working party on the application of economic principles to health service management*, King Edward's Hospital Fund for London, Foreword.

Chapter 2

1 H. C. Cameron (1954) *Mr Guy's Hospital 1726–1948*, London: Longmans, p. 55.

2 Cameron, *Mr Guy's Hospital*, p. 89.

3 For a discussion about the ways in which local social, political, and economic factors combine with medical education to produce specific 'forms of institutional life' in different places see T. N. Bonner (1995) *Becoming a Physician: Medical Education in Britain, France, Germany, and the United States, 1750–1945*, Oxford: Oxford University Press, p.11.

4 (1968) *History of Nursing 1725–1968*, Guy's Hospital Nursing League: NCH Printing.

5 Cameron, *Mr Guy's Hospital*, p. 339.

6 Cameron, *Mr Guy's Hospital*, pp. 362–3. For an account of how heart surgery developed at Guy's through the Peacock Club see T. Treasure (2017) *The Heart Club: A history of London's heart surgery pioneers*, London: Clink Street Publishing.

7 Cameron, *Mr Guy's Hospital*, p. 400. See also J. E. Pater (1981) *The Making of the National Health Service*, London: King Edward's Hospital Fund for London, pp.24-25.

8 Cameron, *Mr Guy's Hospital*, p. 464.

9 Teaching hospitals, in particular, benefited from the EMS funding arrangements. See M. Lambert (2011) 'The virtues of decentralisation for health services in crisis', *History & Policy*, Policy Paper [online] Available at: http://www.historyandpolicy. org/policy-papers/papers/the-virtues-of-decentralisation-forhealth-services-in-crisis [Accessed 15 Aug 2023].

10 Cameron, *Mr Guy's Hospital*, p. 389.

11 R. Sharpington (1980) *Towards Improved Health Care. No Substitute for the Governors. 50 years in the management and administration of St Thomas' Hospital 1927-1977,* London, p.28.

12 C. Webster (1988) *The Health Services since the War: Volume I. Problems of Health Care. The National Health Service Before 1957*, London: HMSO, p. 122.

13 Sharpington, *Towards Improved Health Care*, p. 63.

14 Interview with Joachim Jose, 17 December 2013.

15 Interview with Barbara Stevens, 17 December 2013.

16 Author correspondence with Luis and Krystyna Ribeiro.

17 B. McSwiney (2008) 'Down Memory Lane', *The Veteran: The newsletter for veterans of Guy's and St Thomas'*, Issue 44, Summer, p.6.

18 Bryan's initiative chimed with the policies of the time which were moving to a position where teaching hospitals 'should act as district general hospitals, the students being taught where the patients required treatment – not vice versa.' G. Rivett (1986) *The Development of the London Hospital System 1823-1982*, London: King Edwards' Hospital Fund For London, p.292.

19 Sharpington, *Towards Improved Health Care* p. 44.

20 W. Holland (2013) *Improving Health Services: Background, Method and Applications*, Cheltenham: Edward Elgar, p.115. The Unit's publications included: G. McLachlan (ed.) (1971) *Portfolio for Health: The Role and Programme of the Department of Health and Social Security in Health Service Research,* London: Nuffield Provincial Hospitals Trust/Oxford University Press and G. McLachlan (ed.) (1971) *Portfolio for Health 2: The Developing Programme of the Department of Health and Social Security,*

London: Nuffield Provincial Hospitals Trust/Oxford University Press. See also W. Holland and J. W. Owen (1974) 'A Conflict of Roles', *Health and Social Service Journal*, 16 March.

21 S. Sheard (2014) *The Passionate Economist: How Brian Abel-Smith shaped global health and social welfare*, Bristol: Policy Press, p. 133.

22 Sharpington, *Towards Improved Health Care*, p. 45

23 Sharpington, *Towards Improved Health Care*, p. 45.

24 JWO St Thomas' Health District (n.d) *District Profile*, p. 50.

25 JWO St Thomas' Hospital (1966) *Current Affairs for the Information of Staff*, vol 66 issue no 7, p.262.

26 Sharpington, *Towards Improved Health Care*, p. 43.

27 Sharpington, *Towards Improved Health Care*, p. 43.

28 For details of the training scheme see P. Begley (2020) '"The type of person needed is one possessing a wide humanity": the development of the NHS national administrative training scheme', *Contemporary British History*, vol 34 issue 2, pp.228-250 and S. J. Snow (2013) "'I've Never Found Doctors to Be a Difficult Bunch': Doctors, Managers and NHS Reorganisations in Manchester and Salford, 1948–2007" *Medical History* vol 57 issue 1, pp.65–86.

29 G. Schuster (1959) 'Creative Leadership in a State Service', in The Acton Society Trust, *Hospitals and the State: Hospital Organisation and Administration under the National Health Service: The Impact of Change*, London: Acton Society Trust, 1956–59, 6 volumes, vol 6, p.37.

30 Interview with Richard Sawyer, 27 September 2012.

31 Interview with John Wyn Owen, 30 November 2012.

32 G. L. Davies (1972) 'Why Guy's?' *Guy's Hospital Gazette*, Centenary Edition, 1872–1972, p.62 and p.119.

33 Lost Hospitals of London: Dunoran House. [online] Available at: https://ezitis.myzen.co.uk/dunoran.html - [Accessed 19 Aug 2023].

34 Interview with Sandra Carnall Ferrelly, 26 September 2012.

35 A. Flexner (1910) *Medical Education in the United States and Canada: A Report to the Carnegie Foundation for the Advancement of Teaching*, New York City: Carnegie Foundation.

36 Ministry of Health (1944) *Report of the Inter-Departmental Committee on Medical Schools*, London: HMSO, pp. 8-9 and

p.11. See also K. Waddington (2003) *Medical Education at St Bartholomew's Hospital 1123– 1995,* Woodbridge, Boydell Press p. 282; G. Rivett (1997) *From Cradle to Grave: Fifty years of the NHS,* London: King's Fund, pp.97-99.

37 By the end of the First World War, seven of the London medical schools accepted women although neither Guy's nor St Thomas' were among these. But as male students returned from the War, prejudice against women students built, especially from male Oxbridge students who came to London to undertake their clinical studies and women were again excluded from training. The issues around the admission of women in the case of St Mary's is discussed in E. Heaman (2003) *St Mary's: The history of a London teaching hospital*, Canada: McGill-Queen's University Press, pp.245-50.

38 Royal Commission (1968) *Report on Medical Education* 1965–68 (Chairman: Lord Todd) Cmnd 3569, London: HMSO.

39 H. Oakeley (ed.) (2010) *St Thomas' Hospital Medical School: The year of 1960, 50 years on*, Beckenham: H. Oakeley, p. 87.

40 Interview with Dundas Moore, 17 September 2013.

41 Interview with Richard Hughes, 22 April 2013.

42 For a discussion of the struggle to establish high quality clinical training in Oxford see C. Webster (1994) 'Medicine', in B. Harrison (ed.) (1994) *The History of the University of Oxford: Volume VIII: The Twentieth Century*, Oxford: Oxford University Press, pp.317-343.

43 Interview with Cyril Chantler, 16 September 2013.

44 Waddington, *Medical education at St Bartholomew's Hospital*, p. 304.

45 Waddington, *Medical education at St Bartholomew's Hospital*, p. 307.

46 Interview with Penny Hewitt, 6 March 2014.

47 The ratio of applicants to places stood at 19:1 for men, 40:1 for women and 100:1 for overseas students. Oakeley, *St Thomas' Hospital Medical School.*

48 Oakeley, *St Thomas' Hospital Medical School*, p.31.

49 Interview with Peter Christie, 30 August 2013.

50 Interview with Hywel Thomas, 13 December 2013.

51 Interview with Tim Clark, 14 June 2013.

52 Interview with Alan Maryon Davis, 13 December 2013.

53 Interview with Tina Challacombe, 5 February 2014.
54 I. Cameron (2019) 'Stephen Semple obituary', *The Guardian*, 20 February.
55 Interview with Ian Cameron, 28 August 2013.
56 Interview with David Barlow, 30 August 2013.
57 Interview with 002.
58 Interview with Cyril Chantler, 16 September 2013.
59 Interview with Alan Maryon Davis, 13 December 2013.
60 Interview with Richard Hughes, 22 April 2013.
61 Interview with Tina Challacombe, 5 February 2014.
62 Interview with Penny Hewitt, 6 March 2014.
63 J. Davenport (1985) 'A Worm's Eye View of the Anaesthetic Department', in Joseph Rupreht *et al* (eds), *Anaesthesia – Essays on its History*, Berlin: Springer-Verlag, pp. 357–60.
64 Interview with Barry Jackson, 12 June 2013.
65 A. Howard (2010) *Guy's Hospital Nurses' League 1900–2010*, London, p. xiv.
66 Sister Thirza (1972) 'The School of Nursing 1945–72', *Guy's Hospital Gazette: Centenary Edition 1982-1972*, p. 89.
67 Guy's and St Thomas' NHS Foundation Trust (2018) 'Nurse returns to St Thomas' Hospital over 65 years after training there', 13 March. [online] Available at: https://www.guysandstthomas.nhs.uk/news/nurse-returns-st-thomas-hospital-over-65-years-after-training-there [Accessed 19 Aug 2023].
68 Interview with Kay Riley, 17 September 2013.
69 Author correspondence with Caroline Cave née Jackson.
70 Interview with Deborah Hofman, 24 April 2014.
71 Interview with Francis Tibbles, 13 December 2013.
72 Interview with Betsy Morley, 9 November 2012.
73 Interview with Kay Riley, 17 September 2013.
74 Interview with Alan Maryon Davis, 13 December 2013.
75 Interview with Stephen Challacombe, 5 February 2014.
76 Interview with 002.
77 Interview with Penny Hewitt, 6 March 2014.
78 Interview with Tim Clark, 14 June 2013.
79 Interview with Alan Maryon Davis, 13 December 2013.

Chapter 3

[1] JWO PA Management Consultants (1973) *Report*, MAN/10, Appendix XI.

[2] Snow, *The recent history of Guy's and St Thomas'*, p.17.

[3] N. C. Rogers (1976) 'Clinical Superintendent' in C. Handler (ed.) (1976) *Guy's Hospital: 250 Years*, Guy's Hospital Gazette, pp.231-2. Historically, local authority hospitals were managed by medical superintendents but after the establishment of the NHS in 1948 these posts declined rapidly and were replaced by lay administrators. The medical superintendent post was retained in Scotland and in mental hospitals. Greer's comparative study of England, Scotland and Wales shows that the continuation of this role in Scotland enabled the medical profession to hold fast to significant power in the health system. S. Greer (2004) *Territorial Politics and Health Policy: UK Health Policy in Comparative Perspective*, Manchester: Manchester University Press.

[4] Interview with John Wyn Owen, 30 November 2012. Management consultants had begun advisory work in hospitals since at least the 1950s. See P. Begley and S. Sheard (2019) 'McKinsey and the "Tripartite Monster": The Role of Management Consultants in the 1974 NHS Reorganisation', *Medical History* vol 63(4) pp.390-410, p.398.

[5] Sir George Edward Godper, Chief Medical Officer of Health, 1960-1973.

[6] WT PP/DSC/B/3/4, Letter from Dr C. L. Joiner to David Stafford Clark, 10 April 1984.

[7] Interview with Patricia Moberly, 23 August 2012.

[8] Snow, *The recent history of Guy's and St Thomas'*, p.22.

[9] Sharpington, *Towards Improved Health Care*, p.1.

[10] David Stafford-Clark was a psychiatrist and Director of the York Clinic at Guy's Hospital. He was commissioned to research and write a history of Guy's hospital and he titled the draft, *The Guy's Story: Personality of a Hospital*. The history was never completed nor published because of a dispute with the Trustees who were funding the work. Stafford-Clark's notes and drafts are archived at the Wellcome Trust PP/DSC/B/3/4.

[11] The planning process was impeded by the slow release of key information by the Department of Health and Social Security.

In December 1973, St Thomas' was still waiting for information on capital and revenue expenditure, budgetary control and the organisation of paramedical work. JWO PA Management Consultants (1973) *St Thomas' Hospital: Restructuring the Administrative Organisation*, Report OS 1, December, Appendix V.

[12] Under the 1973 NHS Reorganisation Act, the endowment funds held by teaching and university hospitals were put under the control of special trustees, appointed by the Secretary of State for Health.

[13] WT PP/DSC/B/3/4 Stafford-Clark chapter draft.

[14] WT PP/DSC/B/3/4 Stafford-Clark chapter draft.

[15] Snow, *The recent history of Guy's and St Thomas'*, p.15.

[16] Interview with Peter Lumsden, 7 September 2012.

[17] Snow, *The recent history of Guy's and St Thomas'*, p.32. See also LMA H01/WL/A12/1-2, Special Trustees for St Thomas' Hospital, Report for 1977/78 and 1978/79.

[18] E. M. McInnes (1990) *St Thomas' Hospital*, London: Special Trustees for St Thomas' Hospital, 2nd ed. p.200.

[19] Interview with Patricia Mowbray, 5 September 2012.

[20] Author correspondence with Patricia Mowbray.

[21] SCF *Guylines: Staff Bulletin of the Guy's Group of Hospitals*, No. 21, December 1973, pp.7-9.

[22] SCF *Guylines: Staff Bulletin of the Guy's Group of Hospitals*, No. 21, December 1973, pp.7-9.

[23] Snow, *The recent history of Guy's and St Thomas'*, p.32

[24] Interview with 001. NT Briefing Paper (1981) *The Special Trustees* 10 March. The Paper notes that endowment funds produce an income of a little over £3m per year and assets were split across portfolios of stock exchange investments, farm properties and urban properties.

[25] Interview with John Wyn Owen, 30 November 2012.

[26] Interview with Marcel Jacquemin, 8 March 2013.

[27] Interview with John Wyn Owen, 30 November 2012.

[28] J. Wyn Owen and F. W. Draper (1976) 'Management education, training and development', *Hospital and Health Services Review*, September, pp.301-303.

[29] JWO J. Wyn Owen (2008) *Health Futures: The challenges for Academic Medical and Health Science Centres*, 18 July. Text of speech.

30 O. Rassam (1976) 'Hospital Adopts Business Management Techniques', *International Management*, November, pp.29-31.

31 Interview with Gwyn Williams, 4 July 2013.

32 R. J. Robinson (1976) 'Teaching of Paediatrics at Guy's Hospital', in C. Handler (ed.) *Guy's Hospital: 250 Years*, Guy's Hospital Gazette, p.173.

33 Interview with Cyril Chantler, 16 September 2013.

34 S. M. Crowther, L. A. Reynolds, E. M. Tansey (eds) (2009) *History of Dialysis, c.1950-1980: Wellcome Witnesses to Twentieth Century Medicine*, London: Wellcome Trust Centre for the History of Medicine, vol 37.

35 Interview with Cyril Chantler, 16 September 2013.

36 Interview with Natalie Tiddy, 4 July 2013.

37 Interview with Richard Thompson, 31 March 2014.

38 In 1970 the Lewin Report recommended the introduction of a new grade of staff in operating theatres called operating department assistants. (1970) *The Organisation and Staffing of Operating Departments: A Report of a Joint Sub-Committee*, London: HMSO.

39 Interview with Eddyna Danso, 11 December 2012.

40 W. T. Brown (1978) 'Owed to the Nightingale', *Nursing Times*, 3 August, pp.1273-8.

41 R. Brock (1976) 'Oration', in C. Handler (ed.) (1976) *Guy's Hospital: 250 Years*, Guy's Hospital Gazette, pp.16-31, p.29.

42 Ibid, p.31.

43 Ibid, p.21.

44 C. Handler (ed.) (1976) *Guy's Hospital: 250 Years*, Guy's Hospital Gazette, p.13.

45 RS St Thomas' Hospital (1976) North Wing Opening Brochure, p.2

46 G. Wetherly-Mein (1977) 'The Opening of the New North Wing', *St Thomas' Hospital Gazette*, vol 75 no 1, p.8.

47 King Edward's Hospital Fund for London, *Accounting for Health*.

48 Snow, *The recent history of Guy's and St Thomas'*, p.17.

49 M. Gorsky and G. Millward (2018) 'Resource Allocation for Equity in the British National Health Service, 1948–89: An Advocacy Coalition Analysis of the RAWP', *J Health Polit Policy Law* 1 February vol 43 issue 1, pp.69–108, p.82.

50 Snow, *The recent history of Guy's and St Thomas'*, pp.19-22. See also J. M. Forsythe (1977) 'Philanthropic Organisations and the NHS', *British Medical Journal*, 1 January, p.61. During the 1960s

and 1970s there was a succession of inquiries into the poor conditions in mental hospitals including Ely Hospital (1969), the Whittingham Hospital (1972) and South Ockendon Hospital (1974) which provided evidence of poor nursing and medical care, ill-treatment, and cruelty to patients. See J. P. Martin (with D. Evans) (1984) *Hospitals in Trouble*, Oxford: Basil Blackwell.

51 M. Gorsky and V. Preston (eds) (2014) *The Resource Allocation Working Party: Origins, Implementation and Development, 1974-1990*, Institute of Contemporary British History and London School of Hygiene and Tropical Medicine.

52 *Daily Telegraph* (1976) Friday 26 November, Front and back page.

53 Interview with Ron Kerr, 5 February 2014. For an analysis of the changing nature of politics and local community in Southwark see S. Goss (1988) *Local Labour and Local Government: A study of changing interests, politics and policy in Southwark, 1919 to 1982*, Edinburgh: Edinburgh University Press.

54 Interview with Barry Jackson, 12 June 2013.

55 Interview with Cyril Chantler, 16 September 2013.

56 Interview with Patricia Moberly, 23 August 2012.

57 Interview with Barry Jackson, 12 June 2013.

58 JWO Leeds Castle File, Strategies Workshop, Introduction.

59 These schemes increased allocations to regions to recompense for anticipated spending on new building under the Hospital Plan. See M. Gorsky and G. Millward, 'Resource Allocation for Equity.'

60 Editorial (1979) 'Cash limits squeeze in London AHA(T)s', *British Medical Journal*, 15 December, p.1600.

61 Lambeth, Southwark and Lewisham Area Health Authority, Hansard, 23 October 1979; Lambeth, Southwark and Lewisham Area Health Authority, Hansard, 26 February 1980 [online] Available at: https://api.parliament.uk/historic-hansard/commons/1980/feb/26/lambeth-southwark-and-lewisham-area - [Accessed 19 Aug 2023]. See also J. Lister (1979) 'Cash Limits and the Rebels of Lambeth', *The New England Journal of Medicine*, 1 November, p.984.

62 Interview with Barry Jackson, 12 June 2013.

63 TNA PREM 19/301. Letter dated 29 February 1980 from D. Brereton, Department of Health and Social Security to Nick Sanders, Private Secretary to the Prime Minister.

64 McInnes, *St Thomas' Hospital*, pp.192-3.

65 Snow, *The recent history of Guy's and St Thomas'*, pp.35-6 and author correspondence with Liz Jenkins, 26 June 2011.
66 Interview with Wyndham Lloyd-Davies, 17 December 2014.
67 Interview with Norman Jones. [online] Available at: https://rcp. soutron.net/Portal/Default/en-GB/RecordView/Index/61800 [Accessed 19 Aug 2023].
68 Interview with Wyndham Lloyd-Davies, 17 December 2014.
69 Interview with Marianne Vennegoor, 4 December 2013.
70 Interview with Brian Marchant, 4 April 2013.
71 Interview with Francis Tibbles, 13 December 2013.
72 JWO W. Holland, R. J. Maxwell, J. Wyn Owen (1978) Submission to the Royal Commission on the National Health Service, 'Not Panaceas, but Signposts', 14 April.

Chapter 4

1 api.parliament.uk. (n.d.). *National Health Service (Hansard, 18 February 1982)*. [online] Available at: https://api.parliament.uk/ historic-hansard/commons/1982/feb/18/national-health-service [Accessed 12 August 2023].
2 Snow, *The recent history of Guy's and St Thomas'*, p.30.
3 *Circle: The Magazine for the West Lambeth Health Authority (Circle)*, Issue 2, 1982, p.3-4
4 *Circle*, Issue 1, 1982, pp.2-3.
5 Snow, *The recent history of Guy's and St Thomas'*, pp.27-28.
6 Ibid.
7 For more details see 'Interview with Ted Knight' in *Marxism Today*, 1981, pp.11-15. [online] Available at: https://banmarchive.org.uk/ marxism-today/january-1981/ted-knight-interview/ [Accessed 19 Aug 2023]
8 Snow, *The recent history of Guy's and St Thomas'*, p.30.
9 Interview with Patricia Moberly, 23 August 2012.
10 Interview with Elaine Murphy, 19 June 2013.
11 *Circle*, Issue 3, 1982, p.2.
12 Nuffield Trust. (n.d.). G. Rivett, *The History of the NHS, 1978–1987: Clinical advance and financial crisis*. [online] Available at: https://www.nuffieldtrust.org.uk/chapter/1978-1987-clinical-advance-and-financial-crisis#toc-header-8 [Accessed 20 Nov. 2023].

[13] Interview with Lee Soden, 8 March 2013.

[14] JL Health Emergency (1984) *The Bulletin of London Health Emergency* no 1 April.

[15] The problems of escalating healthcare costs were not confined to the UK. The US and Europe were also struggling to manage revenue declines and increased demand. For the US see J. P. Swazey (2012) *Merger Games: The Medical College of Pennsylvania, Hahnemann University, and the Rise and Fall of the Allegheny Health Care System*, Philadelphia: Temple Publishing, pp.28-30.

[16] F. Dainton (1982) *Reflections on the Universities and the National Health Service*, Nuffield Provincial Hospitals Trust, pp.154-5.

[17] Dainton, *Reflections,* p.151.

[18] For discussion of the Flowers' report and the consequences for other London teaching hospitals see H. Gay (2007) *The History of Imperial College London 1907-2007*, London: Imperial College Press.

[19] See Chapter 2 note 38.

[20] KCLA Notes on Flowers Report TH/AD12/32. See also *The Lancet* (1980) 15 November, pp.1091-1093.

[21] Interview with Tim Matthews, 27 August 2013.

[22] Interview with Tim Clark, 14 June 2013.

[23] Nuffield Trust. (n.d.). G. Rivett, *The History of the NHS, 1978–1987: Clinical advance and financial crisis*. [online] Available at: https://www.nuffieldtrust.org.uk/chapter/1978-1987-clinical-advance-and-financial-crisis#toc-header-8 [Accessed 2 May 2021].

[24] B. Creamer (1986) 'History Q.S.', *St Thomas' Hospital Gazette*, Summer, pp.3-5. Brian Creamer, gastroenterologist and St Thomas' alumnus, was appointed Dean of the Medical School in 1979. His work focused on movement disorders of the gullet and he established the dynamic turnover of intestinal cells in coeliac disease. Donations from Lord Rayne supported the creation of an 'extensive research floor' and the gastroenterology unit moved there in 1976. Whilst Dean, Creamer fundraised for a new student hostel in the ground of Lambeth Palace which is named after him. Richard Thompson (2005) 'Brian Creamer Obituary,' *British Medical Journal* vol 331 15 October, p.909.

25 SC S. Challacombe and R. Watson (n.d.) *Merger of Guy's and KCH Dental Schools: Establishing the Dental Institute.*
26 Interview with Ian Gainsford, 7 November 2012.
27 B. Creamer, 'History Q.S.'.
28 Interview with Barry Jackson, 12 June 2013.
29 Interview with Richard Thompson, 31 March 2014.
30 Interview with Ian Cameron, 28 August 2013.
31 B. Creamer, 'History Q.S.'.
32 005 Interviewee
33 Interview with Elaine Murphy, 19 June 2013.
34 Interview with Hywel Thomas, 13 December 2013.
35 Interview with Stephen Challacombe, 5 February 2014.
36 Interview with Jangu Banatvala, 6 September 2012.
37 Interview with Ian Gainsford, 7 November 2012.
38 Anon (n.d.) *Memoirs*. Personal papers shared with author.
39 *Circle*, Issue 2, 1990, p.4.
40 Interview with David Barlow, 20 August 2013.
41 Interview with David Barlow, 20 August 2013.
42 *St Thomas' Hospital Gazette* (1989) Spring, p.43.
43 Interview with Jangu Banatvala, 6 September 2012.
44 Interview with Tony Gardner, 31 August 2013.
45 *Sunday Observer* (1984) 4 March, p.16.
46 *Guardian* (1984) 7 March, p.5.
47 M. Gorsky (ed.) (2010) *The Griffiths NHS Management Inquiry: its origins, nature and impact*, Witness Seminar, held 11th November 2008, Centre for History in Public Health, London School of Hygiene and Tropical Medicine. [online] Available at https://www.lshtm.ac.uk/media/31881 - [Accessed 20 Aug 2023].
48 Interview with Peter Griffiths, 10 June 2013.
49 Interview with Cyril Chantler, 16 September 2013.
50 C. Chantler (1990) 'Management Reform in a London Hospital', in N. Carle (ed.) (1990) *Managing for Health Result*, London: King Edward's Hospital Fund for London, p.76. See also C. Chantler (1993) 'Historical background: where have clinical directorates come from and what is their purpose?', in A. Hopkins (ed.) (1993) *The Role of Hospital Consultants in Clinical Directorates*, London: Royal College of Physicians, pp.1-103.
51 CC C. Chantler (2012) *Modern Medicine and the National Health Service: Lecture to the University of Kent*, 27 January.

52 Interview with Jeremy Brinley Codd, 17 December 2013.

53 Chantler (1990) 'Management Reform', p.80.

54 C. Chantler (1999) 'The role and education of doctors in the delivery of health care', *Lancet* 3 April, pp.1178-81.

55 Chantler (1993) 'Historical background', p.10.

56 *Circle*, Issue 1, 1980, p.1 and Issue 3, 1981, p.9.

57 Anon, *Memoirs*, personal papers shared with author.

58 Interview with 006.

59 RS (1986) Memo, Proposals for Cuts in 1986/87, RSS/ECM 27 March.

60 *Circle*, Issue 1, 1987, p.1.

61 *St. Thomas's Hospital (Hansard, 27 November 1987)*. [online] Available at: https://api.parliament.uk/historic-hansard/commons/1987/nov/27/st-thomass-hospital [Accessed 8 August 2023].

62 CC Letter to Cyril Chantler, 12 November 1987.

63 Dr Graham Winyard in *The NHS Internal Market Witness Seminar*, held on 5 December 2017 at the University of Liverpool in London, published by the Department of Public Health and Policy, University of Liverpool, 2018, p.23.

64 Interview with Jeremy Brinley Codd, 17 December 2013.

65 In 1966, St Thomas' had been one of the few hospitals to introduce a compressed two-year nurse training course for girls with university degrees. *Sunday Telegraph* (1966) 11 September, p.32.

66 E. L. Jones and S. J. Snow (2010) *Against the Odds: Black, Minority and Ethnic Clinicians and Manchester*, Carnegie Publishing: Manchester NHS Primary Care Trust and The Centre For the History of Science, Technology and Medicine, p.54.

67 Interview with Eddyna Danso, 11 December 2012.

68 See A. Beach and C. Davies (2000) *Interpreting Professional Self-Regulation: A History of the United Kingdom Central Council for Nursing, Midwifery and Health Visiting*, London: Routledge.

69 C. Davies (1995) *Gender and the professional predicament in nursing*, Buckingham: Open University Press. Nuffield Trust. (n.d.). G. Rivett, *The History of the NHS, 1978–1987: Clinical advance and financial crisis*. [online] Available at: https://www.nuffieldtrust.org.uk/chapter/1978-1987-clinical-advance-and-financial-crisis#toc-header-8 [Accessed 2 May 2021].

70 TH *Guylines: Staff Bulletin of the Guy's Health District*, January/
   February 1981, p.4 and March/April 1981, p.3.
71 Commission on Nursing Education (1985) *The education of
   nurses: a new dimension*, London: Royal College of Nursing.
72 Interview with Eddyna Danso, 11 December 2012.
73 Interview with 009.
74 Interview with Hywel Thomas, 13 December 2013.
75 JL (1987) *Bulletin of London Health Emergency* No.15, April, p.8.
76 Interview with Graham Haynes, 13 December 2013.
77 Interview with Patricia Moberly, 23 August 2012.
78 Interview with Helen Lewis, 3 April 2014.
79 PM Notes on recollections.
80 Snow, *The recent history of Guy's and St Thomas'*, p.35.
81 Interview with Natalie Tiddy, 4 July 2013.
82 Interview with Mike Messer, 8 November 2012.
83 For the longer history of the Nightingale School and the changes
   driven by *Project 2000* see Roy Wake (1983) *The Nightingale
   Training School 1860-1996*, London: Haggerston Press.
84 Interview with Graham Haynes, 13 December 2013.
85 The Nightingale and Guy's College of Health (1993) *Education for
   Healthcare in the 21st Century*.
86 A. Howard (2010) *Guy's Hospital: Nurses' League, 1900-2000*,
   London: Guy's Nurses Hospital League, p.87.
87 Interview with 012.
88 Author correspondence with Sue Norman.
89 Interview with Natalie Tiddy, 4 July 2013.
90 Interviews with Hywel Thomas; Alan Maryon Davis; Graham
   Haynes, 13 December 2014.
91 Interview with Tina Challacombe, 5 February 2014
92 *Circle*, Issue 3, 1983, p.2.
93 Admin (n.d.). *Our Collections*. [online] Florence Nightingale
   Museum London. Available at: https://www.florence-nightingale.
   co.uk/history-of-the-collection/. [Accessed 21 Apr 2021]
94 F. Candlin (2012) 'Independent museums, heritage and the shape
   of museum studies' *Museums & Society* vol 10 March pp.28-41.
95 PM Notes on recollections.
96 PM Notes on recollections. Patricia was later awarded an MBE in
   recognition of her work on the Museum.

[97] PM (n.d.) The Florence Nightingale Museum Trust, Events Committee: Record of Events 1984 to 1999.

[98] Interview with Natalie Tiddy, 4 July 2013.

[99] Interview with Natalie Tiddy, 4 July 2013.

[100] Chantler, 'The role and education of doctors'.

[101] T. Bate, D. G. Clarke, A. M. Hoy, P. P. Laird (1981) 'The St Thomas' Hospital Terminal Care Support Team: A New Concept of Hospice Care', *The Lancet*, 30 May, pp.1201-1203.

[102] Author correspondence with Thelma Bates.

[103] V. Berridge (1999) *Health and Society in Britain since 1939*, Cambridge: Cambridge University Press, p.73.

[104] Interview with Rupert Whitaker, 19 June 2013.

[105] www.tht.org.uk. (2022). *How it all began | Terrence Higgins Trust*. [online] Available at: https://www.tht.org.uk/our-work/about-our-charity/our-history/how-it-all-began. [Accessed 1 May 2021]

[106] Interview with David Barlow, 30. August 2013.

[107] Interview with Rupert Whitaker, 19 June 2013.

[108] Interview with Helen Lewis, PhD, MSc Biochemistry, 3 April 2012. The research was published, see H. Lewis and S. Arber (2015) 'Impact of age at onset for children with renal failure on education and employment transitions', *Health*, vol 19, no 1, (January), pp. 67–85.

[109] The Nuffield Trust. (2019). G. Rivett, *The History of the NHS, 1988–1997: New influences and new pathways*. [online] Available at: https://www.nuffieldtrust.org.uk/chapter/1988-1997-new-influences-and-new-pathways. [Accessed 20 April 2021]

[110] T. Butcher, (1995) 'A New Civil Service? The Next Steps Agencies' in R Pyper and L Robins (eds) (1995) *Governing the UK in the 1990s*, London: Palgrave, pp.61-81.

[111] Interview with Karen Caines, 4 June 2014.

[112] Interview with Elaine Murphy, 19 June 2013.

[113] Butterworths Medico-Legal Reports/Volume 10/R v Secretary of State for Health and others, ex parte Keen - 10 BMLR 13.

[114] Interview with Peter Griffiths, 10 June 2013. Ian McColl, Baron McColl of Dulwich, CBE (b. 1933), Professor of Surgery at Guy's Hospital and Shadow Minister for Health, 1997-2000.

[115] Interview with Maurice Lessof, 16 December 2013.

116 National Audit Office (1998) *Cost Over-runs, Funding Problems and Delays on Guy's Hospital Phase III Development*, HC 761 Session 1997-98.,Department of Health, 18 June, p.7. webarchive.nationalarchives.gov.uk. (n.d.). *UK Government Web Archive*. [online] Available at: https://webarchive. nationalarchives.gov.uk/ukgwa/20170207054802/https://www. nao.org.uk/pubsarchive/wp-content/uploads/sites/14/2018/11/ Department-of-Health-Cost-Over-runs-Funding-Problems-and-Delays-on-Guys-Hospital-Phase-III-Development.pdf [Accessed 20 Nov. 2023].

117 Interview with Philip Harris, 11 September 2012.

118 Interview with Karen Caines, 4 June 2014.

119 Interview with Karen Caines, 4 June 2014.

120 Interview with Wilma MacPherson, 21 February 2013.

121 (1991) 'Guy's and Lewisham Trust sorts itself out', *British Medical Journal*, 4 May, p.1039.

122 Interview with Karen Caines, 4 June 2014.

123 (1991) *Hospital Doctor*, 2 May.

124 Interview with Peter Griffiths, 10 June 2013.

125 Interview with Wilma MacPherson, 21 February 2013.

126 Interview with Philip Harris, 11 September 2012.

127 Interview with Lee Soden, 8 March 2013.

128 (1992) *Independent*, 15 December.

129 KC (1992) Memo to all members of the Guy's Management Executive: Guy's Management Philosophy, 5 February.

130 Interview with Karen Caines, 4 June 2014.

131 M. Blume (1991) 'Gourmet Food Where You Least Expect It', *The New York Times*, 29 July.

132 (1990) *St Thomas' Hospital Gazette*, Spring, p.7.

133 *The Times* reported that 52 per cent of a staff turnout of 82 per cent opposed the move to Trust status. 27 February 1990, p.2 By June 1990 the opposition to the proposals had increased to 96 per cent of consultants. *The Times*, 8 June 1990, p.5 and 30 November 1990, p.2.

134 F. Godlee and A. Walker (1990) 'Tale of two hospitals', *British Medical Journal*, vol 301, pp.154-56.

135 *Circle*, March 1993, p.4.

136 As noted earlier, it was becoming common for civil servants from the Department of Health and Social Security who brought

contacts and expertise to take up executive posts in Trusts and Health Authorities. See Day and Klein, and Greer and Jarman, op cit.

[137] In September 1990 the West Lambeth Health Authority had announced cuts of almost £1m to address the anticipated £4.1m deficit that budget year. (1990) *The Times*, 5 September, p.2. *Circle*, Issue 3, 1991, p.2.

[138] WLD Wyndham Lloyd-Davies (1992) 'Care, Cash and Crises: Presidential Address to the British Association of Urological Surgeons.'

Chapter 5

[1] T. Kember and G. Macpherson (1994) *The NHS: A Kaleidoscope of Care – Conflicts of Service and Business Values*, London: Nuffield Provincial Hospital Trust, p.121. See also (1992) King's Fund Commission on the Future of London's Acute Health Services, *London Health Care 2010: Changing the future of services in the capital*, London: King's Fund; S. Sigurgeirsdóttir (2005) *Health Policy and Hospital Mergers: How the impossible became possible*, unpublished PhD thesis, University of London.

[2] B. Tomlinson (1992) *Report of the inquiry into London's health service, medical education and research / Presented to the Secretaries of State for Health and Education by Sir Bernard Tomlinson, London:* HMSO, p.128.

[3] M. Gorsky and V. Preston (eds) (2013) *The Tomlinson Report and After: Reshaping London's Health Services 1992-1997*, Institute of Contemporary History and London School of Hygiene and Tropical Medicine, p.55. Bottomley also reflects on her resolve to take full responsibility for the series of 'very difficult and tough decisions in London' in an interview with Chris Ham. See C. Ham (2000) *The politics of NHS reform 1988-97: metaphor or reality?* London: The King's Fund, p.23.

[4] King's Fund, *London Health Care 2010*; PMob Lord Barney Hayhoe, *Draft speech for National Association of Health Authorities and Trusts Conference*, dated 16 May 1994 but not delivered.

[5] B. Tomlinson, (1992) p.128.

[6] (1993) Department of Health, *Making London Better*, London: HMSO.

7 C. Farrell (1993) *Conflict and Change: Specialist Care in London*, London: King's Fund.
8 Interview with Tim Chessells, 22 April 2014.
9 Interview with 001.
10 Gorsky and Preston (2013) *The Tomlinson Report*.
11 Interview with Karen Caines, 4 June 2014.
12 The Nuffield Trust. (2019). G. Rivett, *The History of the NHS, 1988–1997: New influences and new pathways*. [online] Available at: https://www.nuffieldtrust.org.uk/chapter/1988-1997-new-influences-and-new-pathways. [Accessed 20 April 2021].
13 Interview with John Lister, 11 June 2013.
14 B. Jarman (1993) 'Is London over-bedded?', *British Medical Journal* 10 April, pp.979-982.
15 Interview with Brian Jarman, 26 February 2013.
16 Interview with Brian Jarman, 26 February 2013.
17 Searches on terms such as 'London health reconfiguration' between the dates of 1991 to 1994 at the British Library Newspaper Archive at Colindale produced 1,000s of hits.
18 P Mob Hayhoe, *Draft speech*.
19 Interview with Sandra Carnall Ferrelly, 26 September 2012.
20 Interview with 001.
21 LMA (1992) St Thomas' Hospital, *At the Heart of London's Health*, 8 October. Final submission to the Tomlinson Enquiry Team by St Thomas' Hospital.
22 Interview with Lee Soden, 8 March 2013.
23 Interview with Wilma MacPherson, 21 February 2013.
24 Interview with 001.
25 Interview with Gwyn Williams, 4 July 2013.
26 Interview with Stephen Challacombe, 5 February 2014.
27 Interview with Peter Griffiths, 10 June 2013.
28 *Circle*, March 1993, pp.1-2.
29 Interview with Tim Matthews, 27 August 2013.
30 Interview with 006.
31 TNA UGC 34/21 Letter from John Patten, Secretary of State for Education to Virginia Bottomley, Secretary of State for Health, 17 January 1994.
32 Interview with Simon Hughes, 11 October 2012.
33 Interview with Richard Hughes, 22 April 2013.
34 Interview with Betsy Morley, 9 November 2012.

35 Interview with Michael Gleeson, 29 August 2013.
36 Interview with Malcolm Alexander, 23 August 2012.
37 Interview with Simon Hughes, 11 October 2012.
38 Interview with Maurice Lessof, 16 December 2013.
39 Interview with Simon Hughes, 11 October 2012.
40 Interview with Kay Lucey, 6 September 2012.
41 Interview with Michael Gleeson, 29 August 2013.
42 Interview with Simon Hughes, 11 October 2012.
43 Interview with Wilma MacPherson, 21 February 2013.
44 Interview with Tim Matthews, 27 August 2013.
45 *Circle*, March 1993, p.4.
46 Interview with Tim Matthews, 27 August 2013.
47 Interview with Tim Matthews, 27 August 2013. (1992) St Thomas' Hospital: At the heart of London's health, October.
48 *The Observer Magazine* (1994) 'No Pennies for Guy's', 27 March, p.21.
49 Interview with 006.
50 Interview with John Lister, 11 June 2013.
51 Interview with Marianne Vennegoor, 4 December 2013.
52 Interview with John Pelly, 17 December 2013.
53 Interview with Tim Matthews, 27 August 2013.
54 TNA H09/GY/A/383/002 Guy's and St Thomas' Hospital Trust, *Summary of the Option Appraisal submitted to Virginia Bottomley, Secretary of State for Health*, December 1993.
55 Interview with Tim Matthews, 27 August 2013
56 TNA H09/GY/A/383/002 Guy's and St Thomas' Hospital Trust, *Summary of the Option Appraisal submitted to Virginia Bottomley, Secretary of State for Health*, December 1993.
57 TNA UGC 34/21 Secretary of State's Meeting with Cabinet Colleagues, 1 February 1994: Note on Guy's and St Thomas'.
58 TNA UGC 34/21 Secretary of State's Meeting with Cabinet Colleagues, 1 February 1994: Note on Guy's and St Thomas'.
59 TNA UGC 34/21 Letter from Robert Creighton, Principal Private Secretary, Department of Health to Nick MacPherson, Principal Private Secretary, HM Treasury, 31 January 1994.
60 Interview with 001.
61 TNA UGC 34/21 Letter from Robert Creighton, Principal Private Secretary, Department of Health to Nick MacPherson, Principal Private Secretary, HM Treasury, 31 January 1994.

62 api.parliament.uk. (n.d.). *Health Service (London) (Hansard, 10 February 1994)*. [online] Available at: https://api.parliament.uk/historic-hansard/commons/1994/feb/10/health-service-london [Accessed 21 Nov 2020].

63 *Circle*, March 1993, p.1.

64 Interview with Simon Hughes, 11 October 2012.

65 Interview with Jangu Banatvala, 6 September 2012.

66 Interview with Betsy Morley, 9 November 2012.

67 *Independent* (1995) 'Guy's campaigners lose legal battle', 18 October.

68 The Independent. (1995). *Inside Parliament: Conservatives lose patience as Mrs Bottomley loses*. [online] Available at: https://www.independent.co.uk/news/uk/politics/inside-parliament-conservatives-lose-patience-as-mrs-bottomley-loses-hospitals-1614362.html [Accessed 16 May 2021].

69 Ham, op cit, p.34.

70 Admin (n.d.). *Guy's Hospital (Hansard, 12 December 1997)*. [online] api.parliament.uk. Available at: https://api.parliament.uk/historic-hansard/commons/1997/dec/12/guys-hospital. [Accessed 21 Nov 2020].

71 news.bbc.co.uk. (n.d.). *BBC News | Health | Guy's casualty is closed in £100m reorganisation*. [online] Available at: http://news.bbc.co.uk/1/hi/health/163193.stm [Accessed 20 Aug 2023].

72 Interview with 001.

73 Interview with Richard Hughes, 22 April 2013.

74 (1994) Guy's and St Thomas' Hospital Trust, Statement of the Trust Board, 7 April.

75 PMob Hayhoe, *Draft speech*.

76 Snow, *The recent history of Guy's and St Thomas'*, p.56.

77 Interview with Carole Rowe, 7 March 2014.

78 Interview with Michael Gleeson, 29 August 2013.

79 Interview with Wyndham Lloyd-Davies, 17 December 2013.

80 Interview with 007.

81 Interview with 011.

82 Interview with 011.

83 Interview with 007.

84 Interview with Marianne Vennegoor, 4 December 2013.

85 Interview with Marianne Vennegoor, 4 December 2013.

86 Interview with Marianne Vennegoor, 4 December 2013.

87 Interview with 011.
88 Interview with 007.
89 D. Bihari (1995) Letter to the *Evening Standard*, 3 January, p.41.
90 Interview with 010.
91 Interview with 010.
92 Interview with 006.
93 1996, Save Guy's Campaign Newsletter, February.
94 Interview with Betsy Morley, 9 November 2012.
95 Interview with Neville Smith, 17 September 2013.
96 Interview with John Pelly, 17 December 2013.
97 Interview with John Pelly, 17 December 2013.
98 Anthony Young (2003) *The Medical Manager: A practical guide for clinicians*, London: BMJ Books, 2nd edition, p.224.
99 Interview with 005.
100 National Audit Office (1998) *Cost Over-runs, Funding Problems and Delays on Guy's Hospital Phase III Development*, Department of Health, HC 761 Session 1997-98, 10 June, p.7.
101 SCF Guy's Hospital (1990) Philip Harris House: Information Brochure, July, p.13.
102 The Independent. (1994). *Guy's under new threat*. [online] Available at: https://www.independent.co.uk/news/uk/home-news/guy-s-under-new-threat-1432017.html [Accessed 21 Nov 2020].
103 *The Observer Magazine* (1994) 'No Pennies for Guy's', 27 March, p.21.
104 National Audit Office (1998) *Cost Over-runs*.
105 Interview with Betsy Morley, 9 November 2012.
106 Interview with Alan Maryon Davis, 13 December 2013.
107 Interview with Sandra Carnell Ferrelly, 26 September 2012.
108 Interview with Betsy Morley, 9 November 2012.
109 BM n.d. Compliation of Guy's and St Thomas' Pantomimes.
110 Snow, *The recent history of Guy's and St Thomas'*, p.55.
111 Interview with Betsy Morley, 9 November 2012.
112 Interview with Sandra Carnell Ferrelly, 26 September 2012.
113 Interview with Tim Matthews, 27 August 2013.
114 A. Mold (2015) 'The art of medicine: making British patients into consumers', *The Lancet* vol 385 4 April, pp.1286-1287.

115 B. Edwards and M. Fall (2005) *The Executive Years of the NHS: The England Account 1985-2003*, Oxford: Radcliffe Publishing, pp.100-101.
116 National Audit Office (2001) *Inappropriate adjustments to NHS waiting lists: Report by the Comptroller and Auditor General*, HC452 Session 2001-2002: 19 December, p.14.
117 The Nuffield Trust. (2019). G. Rivett, *The History of the NHS, 1988–1997: New influences and new pathways*. [online] Available at: https://www.nuffieldtrust.org.uk/chapter/1988-1997-new-influences-and-new-pathways. [Accessed 20 April 2021].
118 Interview with Tim Matthews, 27 August 2013.
119 Interview with Michael Cooley, 17 September 2013
120 Interview with Neville Smith, 17 September 2013.
121 Interview with Tim Matthews, 27 August 2013.
122 Virginia Bottomley introduced a policy initiative – Opportunity 2000 – with the aim of increasing the 'quality and quantity of women's participation' in the NHS. See S. Corby (1997) 'Opportunity 2000 in the National Health Service: a missed opportunity for women', *Journal of Management in Medicine* vol 11 no 5, pp.279-293.
123 Interview with Patricia Moberly, 23 August 2012.
124 SCF Guy's and St Thomas' Hospital Trust (1998) *Opening of Thomas Guy House by Her Majesty The Queen*, 18 March.

Chapter 6

1 Heaman op cit, pp.409-10 discusses the case at Imperial College.
2 Interview with Ian Cameron, 28 August 2013.
3 Snow, *The recent history of Guy's and St Thomas'*, p.44.
4 TNA UGC 34/21 Fax from Lord Butterfield, Chairman, UMDS to the Secretary of State for Health and Baroness Julia Cumberlege, 19 January 1994.
5 TNA UGC 34/21 Letter from Rob Hull, Higher Education Funding Council to Shirley Trundle, Department for Education and Employment, 27 October 1995.
6 TNA UGC 34/21 Letter from Rob Hull, Higher Education Funding Council to Shirley Trundle, Department for Education and Employment, 27 October 1995.

7 L .P. Quesne (1987) 'Undergraduate medical education in London: the last 40 years', *Journal of the Royal Society of Medicine*, vol 80, October pp.606-610.

8 Higher Education Funding Council for England (2001) *Increasing medical student numbers in England 2001*.

9 issuu.com. (2009). *KCL-UMDS Merger January 1996 by King's College London - Issuu*. [online] Available at: https://issuu.com/kingscollegelondon/docs/kcl-umds-merger-january-1996 [Accessed 19 Aug 2023].

10 See Swazey, *Merger Games*, chapter 5 for examples of mergers in US teaching hospitals.

11 Interview with Arthur Lucas, 3 July 2013.

12 Author correspondence with Arthur Lucas.

13 Interview with Arthur Lucas, 3 July 2013.

14 Interview with Arthur Lucas, 3 July 2013. See also King's College Act, 1997. Available at: https://www.legislation.gov.uk/ukla/1997/3/enacted [Accessed 19 August 2023].

15 See for example: King's College London Bill Lords (By Order) Volume 280: debated on Monday 24 June 1996 https://hansard.parliament.uk/Commons/1996-06-24/debates [Accessed 19 August 2023].

16 SC Challacombe and Watson, *Merger of Guy's and KCH Dental Schools*.

17 Interview with Gwyn Williams, 4 July 2013.

18 Interview with Gwyn Williams, 4 July 2013.

19 Snow, *The recent history of Guy's and St Thomas'*, pp.49-50.

20 Snow, *The recent history of Guy's and St Thomas'*, p.50.

21 Interview with Stephen Challacombe, 5 February 2014.

22 Interview with David Potter, 6 February 2014.

23 Interview with Gwyn Williams, 4 July 2013.

24 Interview with Gwyn Williams, 4 July 2013.

25 Interview with David Potter, 6 February 2014.

26 Interview with Stephen Challacombe, 5 February 2014.

27 Interview with Hywel Thomas, 13 December 2013.

28 Interview with Gwyn Williams, 4 July 2013.

29 Interview with Gwyn Williams, 4 July 2013.

30 Interview with Gwyn Williams, 4 July 2013.

31 Interview with Gwyn Williams, 4 July 2013.

32 Interview with Arthur Lucas, 3 July 2013.

33 Interview with 001.
34 Interview with Ian Cameron, 28 August 2013.
35 Interview with Hywel Thomas, 13 December 2013.
36 Interview with Gwyn Williams, 4 July 2013.
37 Snow, *The recent history of Guy's and St Thomas'*, p.51.
38 McInnes, *St Thomas' Hospital*, p.199.
39 Interview with John Wyn Owen, 30 November 2012.
40 Interview with Elaine Murphy, 19 June 2013.
41 Interview with Elaine Murphy, 19 June 2013.
42 Interview with Ian Gainsford, 7 November 2012.
43 Interview with 013.
44 LMA Special Trustees of Guy's Hospital, Special Trustees of St Thomas' Hospital, *Briefing Paper to Discuss the Development of a Three-Year Strategy for the Special Trustees*, 21 May 1998.
45 Interview with Geoffrey Shepherd, 1 April 2014.

Chapter 7

1 Interview with Jonathan Michael. [online] Available at https://rcp.soutron.net/Portal/Default/en-GB/RecordView/Index/68043 [Accessed 21 August 2023.]
2 Interview with Patricia Moberly, 23 August 2012.
3 C. Webster (2002). *The National Health Service : a political history*. Oxford ; New York: Oxford University Press, pp.257-8.
4 The Health Foundation (2000). *NHS Plan (2000)*. [online] Policy Navigator. Available at: https://navigator.health.org.uk/theme/nhs-plan-2000 [Accessed 19 August 2023].
5 Admin (n.d.). *'Delivering the NHS Plan: next steps on investment, next steps on reform' report*. [online] Policy Navigator. Available at: https://navigator.health.org.uk/theme/delivering-nhs-plan-next-steps-investment-next-steps-reform-report [Accessed 19 August 2023].
6 Interview with Jonathan Michael.
7 Interview with 001.
8 Interview with Cyril Chantler, 16 September 2013.
9 Snow, *The recent history of Guy's and St Thomas'*, p.65
10 Interview with Dawn Hill, 2 July 2013.
11 Interview with Martin Shaw, 17 December 2013.

12 D. Gaffney, A. M. Pollock, D. Price, and J. Shaoul (1999) 'The private finance initiative: PFI in the NHS---is there an economic case?' *British Medical Journal* vol 319, pp.116–119.

13 Interview with Jonathan Michael.

14 Interview with John Pelly, 17 December 2013. See also K. Palmer and K. Edwards (2011) *Reconfiguring Hospital Services*. London: King's Fund, pp.2-3.

15 Interview with Martin Shaw, 17 December 2013.

16 Admin (n.d.) *New Cancer Centre now open* [online] Guy's and St Thomas' NHS Foundation Trust. Available at: https://www.guysandstthomas.nhs.uk/news/new-cancer-centre-now-open [Accessed 23 August 2023].

17 C. M. Staff (2014). *Essentia outlines plan to offer 'third way' in NHS construction procurement*. [online] Construction Management. Available at: https://constructionmanagement.co.uk/essentia-outlines-plan-offer-third-way-nhs-constru [Accessed 13 May 2023].

18 Population growth and change. (2015). Available at: https://www.lambeth.gov.uk/sites/default/files/ssh-lambeth-population-change-2015-16.pdf [Accessed 19 August 2023].

19 Interview with Mia Hilborn, 3 July 2013.

20 Interview with Comfort Momoh, 5 March 2014.

21 Interview with Patricia Moberly, 23 August 2012.

22 Interview with Eddyna Danso, 11 December 2012.

23 J. M. Simpson, A. Esmail, V. S. Kalra, and S. J. Snow (2010) 'Writing migrants back into NHS history: addressing a 'collective amnesia' and its policy implications', *Journal of the Royal Society of Medicine*, 103(10), pp.392–396, p.393; Jones and Snow, *Against the Odds*.

24 Interview with 008.

25 Interview with 015.

26 Jones and Snow, *Against the Odds*.

27 Interview with 015.

28 Interview with 015.

29 Interview with Bryan Johnson, 4 December 2012.

30 Nuffield Trust (n.d.). G. Rivett, *The History of the NHS 1998–2007: Labour's decade*. [online]. Available at: https://www.nuffieldtrust.org.uk/chapter/1998-2007-labour-s-decade#nursing-education-and-staffing [Accessed 4 July 2021].

31 Interview with Christopher Bramaje and Cecilia Saquing, 6 June 2014.

32 GOV.UK. (2018). *Higher Education Funding Council for England*. [online] Available at: https://www.gov.uk/government/organisations/higher-education-funding-council-for-england.

33 Interview with Rick Trainor, 12 December 2013.

34 See Pamela B Garlick and Gavin Brown (2008) 'Widening participation in medicine', *British Medical Journal*, vol 336, pp.1111-1113. See also Gavin Brown and Pamela B Garlick (2007) 'Changing geographies of access to medical education in London', *Health & Place* 13(2) pp.520-31.

35 Interview with Cyril Chantler, 16 September 2013.

36 Interview with Dawn Hill, 2 July 2013.

37 Interview with Patricia Moberly, 23 August 2012.

38 Interview with Mike Messer, 8 November 2012.

39 Interview with Patricia Moberly, 23 August 2012.

40 Interview with Naveen Cavale, 22 February 2013.

41 Interview with Tina Challacombe, 5 February 2014.

42 Interview with Barry Jackson, 12 June 2013.

43 Interview with Patricia Moberly, 23 August 2012.

44 (n.d.). *Our history | Evelina London*. [online] Available at: https://www.evelinalondon.nhs.uk/about-us/who-we-are/history/our-history.aspx. [Accessed 15 June 2021].

45 Interview with 005.

46 (2015) *The Gist: news from Guy's and St Thomas'*, 'Evelina London celebrates 10 years in its new home', vol 16. [online] Available at: https://www.guysandstthomas.nhs.uk/resources/publications/the-gist/issue-16-the-gist.pdf. [Accessed 15 June 2021].

47 Nuffield Trust (n.d.) G. Rivett, *The History of the NHS, 1998–2007: Labour's decade*. [online] Available at: https://www.nuffieldtrust.org.uk/chapter/1998-2007-labour-s-decade#hospital-building-and-the-private-finance-initiative-pfi [Accessed 17 June 2021].

48 Interview with Dawn Hill, 2 July 2013.

49 Interview with John Pelly, 17 December 2013.

50 Interview with Martin Shaw, 17 December 2013.

51 Zosia Kmietowicz (2005) 'New Children's Hospital for London', *British Medical Journal*, vol 331, p. 1044.

52 Interview with Kay Lucey, 6 September 2012.

53 Interview with Kay Lucey, 6 September 2012.

54 Interview with Bryan Johnson, 4 December 2012.
55 KL (n.d.) Evelina Children's Hospital, Operational and Performance Group: Report on the Staff Focus Groups, p.13.
56 KL (n.d.) Evelina Children's Hospital, Operational and Performance Group: Report on the Staff Focus Groups, p.15.
57 Interview with Dawn Hill, 2 July 2013.
58 Interview with Cyril Chantler, 16 September 2013.
59 Interview with Dawn Hill, 2 July 2013.
60 Interview with Robert Lechler, 1 April 2014.
61 Interview with Robert Lechler, 1 April 2014.
62 Interview with Jawahar, 24 June 2013.
63 Interview with Lewis Moore, 5 May 2014.
64 GKT Gazette (2015) *King's Rebranding GKT is Back*. [online] Available at: https://thegktgazette.wordpress.com/2015/01/07/kings-rebranding-gkt-is-back/ [Accessed 21 August 2023].
65 GKT Gazette, 'King's Rebranding'.
66 Interview with Simon Cleary, 23 April 2014.
67 Interview with Rick Trainor, 12 December 2013.
68 Ismaili.net (n.d.) *Aga Khan's £24m museum bid*. [online] Available at: https://ismaili.net/timeline/2002/20020426tt4.html [Accessed 21 August 2023].
69 C. Blackstock (2002) 'Aga Khan's bid for hospital site rejected'. *The Guardian*. [online] 9 Oct. Available at: https://www.theguardian.com/uk/2002/oct/09/science.highereducation [Accessed 6 August 2023].
70 Interview with Patricia Moberly, 23 August 2012.
71 Interview with Rick Trainor, 12 December 2013.
72 Interview with Robert Lechler, 1 April 2014.
73 Interview with Rick Trainor, 12 December 2013.
74 Interview with Rick Trainor, 12 December 2013.
75 Policy Navigator (n.d.) *'A Framework for Action' review*. [online] Available at: https://navigator.health.org.uk/theme/framework-action-review [Accessed 21 August 2023].
76 Interview with Robert Lechler, 1 April 2014.
77 S. Kitchen (2012) *NHS Guy's and St Thomas' £25m redevelopment, London*. [online] The Architects' Journal. Available at: https://www.architectsjournal.co.uk/competitions/nhs-guys-and-st-thomas-25m-redevelopment-london [Accessed 12 August 2023].

78 Interview with Cyril Chantler, 16 September 2013.

79 The Friends of St Thomas' Hospital, Annual Report 2010/2011, p.31.

Chapter 8

1 Interview with Kay Lucey, 6 September 2012.

2 Interview with Bryan Johnson, 4 December 2012.

3 Interview with Christopher Bramaje and Cecilia Saquing, 6 June 2014.

4 Interview with Mike Messer, 8 November 2012.

5 Interview with Bryan Johnson, 4 December 2012.

6 Interview with Kay Lucey, 6 September 2012.

7 Interview with Kay Lucey, 6 September 2012.

8 The Future Hospital Commission was established by the Royal College of Physicians in 2012 to address growing concerns about the standards of care in hospitals and to recommend improvements. Work at Guy's and St Thomas' was featured in its Case Studies Report. RCP London (2013) *Future Hospital Commission*. [online] Available at: https://www.rcplondon.ac.uk/projects/outputs/future-hospital-commission [Accessed 21 August 2023].

9 Interview with Georgina Day, 5 May 2014.

10 Interview with Georgina Day, 5 May 2014.

11 Interview with Betsy Morley, 9 November 2012.

12 Interview with Georgina Day, 5 May 2014.

13 Bernard M. C. Yam (2013) 'From vocation to profession: the quest for professionalization of nursing', *British Journal of Nursing*, vol 13 no.16 pp.978-982.

14 Interview with Georgina Day, 5 May 2014.

15 Interview with Georgina Day, 5 May 2014.

16 www.kcl.ac.uk (n.d.) *King's Nursing Student wins Student Nursing Times Award 2014 | Website archive | King's College London*. [online] Available at: https://www.kcl.ac.uk/archive/news/nmpc/2014/kings-nursing-student-wins-student-nursing-times-award-2014 [Accessed 21 August 2023].

17 Interview with Richard Thompson, 31 March 2014.

18 Interview with Cyril Chantler, 16 September 2013.

19 Interview with Cyril Chantler, 16 September 2013.

20 Interview with Helen Lawrence, 5 December 2013.
21 M. Taberna, F. Gil Moncayo, E. Jané-Salas *et al*, (2020) The Multidisciplinary Team (MDT) Approach and Quality of Care, *Frontiers in oncology*, 10, 85.
22 General Medical Council (1993) *Tomorrow's Doctors: recommendations on undergraduate medical education*, London.
23 House of Commons Health Committee (24 April 2008) *Modernising Medical Careers* (Third Report of Session 2007–08 Volume I), House of Commons London: The Stationery Office Limited.
24 Interview with Betsy Morley, 9 November 2012.
25 Interview with Cathy Ashley, 11 December 2013.
26 Interview with Patricia Moberly, 23 August 2012.
27 Interview with Francis Tibbles, 13 December 2013.
28 Interview with Ron Kerr, 5 February 2014.
29 Interview with 011; Interview with 014.
30 Interview with Mia Hilborn, 3 July 2013.
31 Interview with 014.
32 Interview with Patricia Moberly, 23 August 2012.
33 Interview with Bryan Johnson, 4 December 2012.
34 Interview with Michael Cooley, 17 September 2013.
35 Interview with Dundas Moore, 17 September 2013.
36 Dundas Moore, 17 September 2013.
37 Interview with Omar Mahroo, 17 September 2013.
38 Interview with 004.
39 Interview with John Bibbings, 8 March 2013.
40 Interview with Comfort Momoh, 5 March 2014.
41 Interview with Christopher Bramaje, 6 June 2014
42 Interview with Cecilia Saquing, 6 June 2014
43 W. Mathews (2009) *My Ward: The story of St Thomas', Guy's and the Evelina Children's Hospitals and their ward names*, London: Walpole House Publishing.
44 Interview with Helen Lawrence, 5 December 2013.
45 Interview with 001.
46 Interview with Eddyna Danso, 11 December 2012.
47 J. A. Seltzer (2019) 'Family Change and Changing Family Demography', *Demography*, vol 56, pp.405-426.
48 Guy's and St Thomas' NHS Foundation Trust. (n.d.). *Guy's and St Thomas' appoints new Chief Nurse*. [online] Available at: https://

www.guysandstthomas.nhs.uk/news/guys-and-st-thomas-appoints-new-chief-nurse [Accessed 18 August 2023].

49 WLD Wyndham Lloyd Davies (1992) 'Care, Cash and Crises: Presidential Address to the British Association of Urological Surgeons.

50 See Pierre Nora's work on sites or realms of memory. P. Nora (1989) 'Between Memory and History: Les Lieux de Mémoire.,' *Representations*, no. 26 pp. 7–24.

Index

Hewitt, Penny 25, 26
Higgins, Terrence 109, 110, 112,
Hilborn, Mia 220, 270, 274
Hill, Dawn 216-7, 222-3, 225,
    229, 235, 240
HIV/Aids 109-113
Hoey, Kate 159
Hofman, Deborah 34
Holland, Walter 16, 43, 60, 72
Hooper, Neil 124
Hopkins, Michael 236
hospitals: administration/
    management 14-9, 41-2,
    49-51, 74, 90-1; bed
    allocation 18; design 17,
    19-22, 33, 108, 176-7, 218,
    236, 237-8, 254; finances/
    financial pressures 7, 11, 51,
    59-64, 72, 73, 74, 124-5, 126,
    142, 190, 200, 216-7, 235,
    284; nursing administration
    53-4, 66; planning 44-5, 49,
    53, 61, 64, 167, 208, 219, 220,
    233, 234, 282
Houses of Parliament 3, 11, 36,
    151, 159
House of Commons 94, 162,
    196
Houston, James (George) 52, 84
Hughes, Richard 24, 29, 152, 163
Hughes, Simon 154-5, 163, 164,
    180, 196
Hurst, Gillian 51

I

Imperial Cancer Research Fund
    177
Imperial College, London 79,
    244, 246, 249
income generation 122-3, 125,
    203, 219
industrial action 39, 59, 77-8
Instant Sunshine 179
intensive care units 68, 92, 163,
    171-2, 225, 236

J

Jackson, Barry 31, 43, 63, 65, 83,
    233
Jacquemin, Marcel 50
Jarman, Brian 144-5
Jawahar, Kaanthan 241-2
Jenkin, Patrick 64-5
Jenkins, Liz 65-6, 102
Jenkins, Stephen 75-6, 126, 263
Johns Hopkins, US 16, 91, 119,
    284
Johnson, Boris 3
Johnson, Bryan 226, 254, 272-3
Jones, Grace 32
Jones, Norman 67, 70
Jose, Joachim 14

K

Keen, Harry 117-8, 121
Kerr, Ron 61-2, 214, 247, 269
King's College Hospital 141, 143
King's College Charity 1

T

Tatton Brown, William 57
Taylor, Hugh 247, 250, 251
technology 79, 168, 172, 190, 228, 253
Thatcher, Margaret 74, 76, 77, 96, 106, 115, 116, 155, 157
Thomas, Hywel 26, 86, 99, 202, 206
Thompson, Richard 55, 83, 261
Tibbles, Francis 34, 70, 268
Tiddy, Natalie 53, 102, 104, 107
Todd report on medical education 23, 80, 189
Tomlinson report on London's health service, medical education and research 139, 140, 141, 144, 146, 147, 150, 156, 157, 159, 162, 191, 209, 281
Trainor, Rick 229, 246
transplants: kidney *see* renal services; blood stem cell 265

U

United Hospitals of the Borough 10, 284
United Friends Hospitals Dining Club 10
United Medical and Dental Schools (UMDS) 7, 82-9, 139, 140, 161-2, 167, 188, 189, 181, 192-207; merger of Guy's and St Thomas' sports

clubs 88, 89, 127; merger with King's College 189-207; merger of UMDS and King's sports clubs 230, 243, 244
urology 126, 168

V

Vauxhall 9, 94, 100, 159
Vennegoor, Marianne 68, 69, 159
Veterans Association 277

W

Waldegrave, Caroline 124
Waldegrave, William 124, 140
Wells, William 193, 194
West Lambeth 50, 58; District Health Authority 74, 75, 76, 77, 88, 94, 125, 126
Wetherly-Mein, G 58
Whitaker, Rupert 109, 110, 112, 113
Winter of Discontent 63
Winyard, Graham 95
Williams, Gwyn 51, 198, 204
Working for Patients, *White Paper* 7, 73, 115
Wright, Nicholas 177
Wyn Owen, John 46, 49-51, 63, 72, 92, 106

Y

Young, Anthony (Tony) 165, 174
Yorke Rosenberg Mardall 17

Printed in Great Britain
by Amazon

57057225R00196